Suicide and Homicide-Suicide Among Police

Antoon A. Leenaars, Ph.D., C.Psych., CPQ
Windsor, Ontario

Death, Value, and Meaning Series
Series Editor: Dale A. Lund

Baywood Publishing Company, Inc.
AMITYVILLE, NEW YORK

Baywood Publishing Company, Inc.
26 Austin Avenue
P.O. Box 337
Amityville, NY 11701
(800) 638-7819
E-mail: baywood@baywood.com
Web site: baywood.com

Library of Congress Catalog Number: 2009051895
ISBN 978-0-89503-390-1 (cloth)
ISBN 978-0-89503-458-8 (epub)
ISBN 978-0-89503-459-5 (epdf)
ISBN 978-0-89503-460-1 (mobi)
http://dx.doi.org/10.2190/SHS

Library of Congress Cataloging-in-Publication Data

Leenaars, Antoon A.
Suicide and homicide-suicide among police / Antoon A. Leenaars.
p. cm. -- (Death, value, and meaning series)
Includes bibliographical references and index.
ISBN 978-0-89503-390-1 (cloth : alk. paper) 1. Police--Suicidal behavior. 2. Police--Mental health. I. Title.
HV7936.S77.L44 2010
362.28088'3632--dc22

2009051895

Suicide in Police at Epidemic Levels.

New York Post, 1934–1940

New York Police Officer Commits Suicide Over Taser Incident

NEW YORK—New York police Lt. Michael Pigott turned 46 on Thursday, but before the sun rose, he slipped out of his home, drove to his former command in Brooklyn and fired a single bullet into his head, police said.

Pigott, a respected 21-year veteran, was declared dead at a hospital. He had been tormented since Sept. 24, when his order to Taser a psychiatric patient led to the man's death, according to police officials and sources.

Several police sources involved in the investigation into the death of Iman Morales, 35, said Pigott was worried that he could lose his job and be indicted. Morales was killed in a 10-foot fall outside his Bedford-Stuyvesant building.

"The lieutenant was deeply distraught and extremely remorseful over the death of Iman Morales in Brooklyn last week," Mayor Michael R. Bloomberg said. "Sadly, his death just compounds the tragedy of the loss of Mr. Morales."

Los Angeles Times, October 3, 2008

Central Falls Police Chief Found Dead At Station

CENTRAL FALLS—Police Chief Thomas Moffatt was found dead of a gunshot in the basement garage of the police station yesterday.

His death appears to have been suicide, according to Rep. Joseph L. Faria, D-Central Falls. Two officers discovered Moffatt's body in his cruiser shortly after 8:30 a.m., Faria said.

Friends and colleagues were stunned, saying Moffatt had the respect of his officers and the city government for turning around a demoralized department. He had just signed his second three-year contract with the city, saying he was happy with his job.

"If there was a list of people you expected to do it, he wouldn't even be on the bottom of the list," said state Sen. Daniel J. Issa, D-Central Falls.

Moffatt, 57, was a 22-year veteran of the state police and was the chief of police in Bristol for eight years before he was appointed in Central Falls in 1995.

"Everybody loved Tommy," said North Smithfield Police Chief Steven E. Reynolds, a former commander of the state police detective division. "He was a great guy. A hell of a trooper."

The Providence Journal, November 21, 1998

Female Officer Pulled Trigger in London, Ont., Murder-Suicide: Police

LONDON, ONT.—It was a murder-suicide that claimed the lives of a retired London, Ont., police superintendent and the force's highest ranking female officer, London police announced Monday.

David Lucio, and Acting Insp. Kelly Johnson were found on Thursday bleeding from gunshot wounds inside a van that crashed into Johnson's downtown apartment building. Johnson, the passenger in the truck, "fired the gunshot that killed David Lucio prior to taking her own life with a single gunshot. As a result, this tragic incident has been determined to be a murder-suicide," Const. Amanda Pfeffer said in a news release.

National Post, June 11, 2007

Dedication

To the survivors; the family, friends, and fellow officers of the 93 officers who died in the great 1930s suicide epidemic in New York, Lieutenant Michael Pigott, Chief Thomas Moffatt, and Superintendent Dave Lucio and Acting Inspector Kelly Johnson

and

To Forensic Psychiatrist Peter Collins and Detective David Gilmore, the best partners one can have in major crime/forensic investigations

and

To Officer Brian Egan, my son-in-law; wellness in officers is a family concern.

Table of Contents

Preface

Suicide is violence. Homicide is violence. Suicide is self-directed violence. Homicide is other-directed violence. They are lethal violence. Suicide, homicide, and when they occur together—homicide-suicide—have probably always been part of human experience. The World Health Organization (WHO, 2002) defines violence as

> The intentional use of physical force or power, threatened or actual, against oneself, another person, or against a group or community, that either results in or has a high likelihood of resulting in injury, death, psychological harm, maldevelopment or deprivation. (p. 5)

It is estimated that 1.6 million people die by violence each year (WHO, 2002). Almost half (800,000) of these are suicides, one third are homicides (530,000) and one-fifth (320,000) are war related. No single factor or event explains why so many people are violent. Violence is multidetermined. Suicide, homicide, and such are the result of an interplay of individual, relationship, social, cultural, and environmental factors. This is sometimes called the ecological model. The model suggests that there are different levels—individual, relationship, community, and societal—that influence suicide and homicide, and thus, by implication, one can prevent behavior at various levels. Explaining suicide and homicide-suicide is one aim of this book.

We plan to outline, for the first time together, the epidemic levels of suicide and homicide-suicide in police. Especially in the media and Internet, high rates in law enforcement officers, such as police, have been reported. This has been less so in the professional literature. There have been a few books, including one by the FBI, but none focus on both suicide and homicide-suicide, showing the latter to be more like a suicide than a homicide. This book begins to explore such questions as: Are rates of suicide in police high? Homicide-suicide? Why do suicides and homicide-suicides occur? Are suicide and homicide related? Why in the police? What are the individual, relational, social, cultural, and environmental factors? Does an emotional disorder (psychopathology) increase risk? Alcoholism? Do police work-stress, divorce, domestic violence, and a multidimensional array of other factors cause risk? What relationship issues are figural? Does the marital situation have an impact? Does the "macho" culture? The "blue" culture? Does the blue culture create barriers, called blue walls? Does the availability of a gun increase risk? In this book, we intend to answer these questions and also to provide some reflections on applications. What is effective in treating police? Can psychotherapy help? And if the officer is suffering work-related Post Traumatic Stress Disorder (PTSD), what is needed? What do police services need to provide? What help is effective? And what are police barriers to wellness? What can police services and communities do? We hope to begin to answer these questions too.

Suicide and homicide-suicide in police are complex, multidetermined events. People, whether a police officer or not, are generally perplexed, stressed, confused, and even overwhelmed when they are confronted by suicide, and even more so by homicide-suicide. The most common response by survivors is "I can't wrap my head around it." Predictive, like suicide, homicide-suicide is difficult to understand. There are at least two reasons: the very complexity of these events and the fact that suicide is a low-frequency event (occurrence) in police, and homicide-suicide in police is also lower (or is it?). There are at least two avenues to understanding: the nomothetic (general) and the idiographic (specific). The nomothetic approach deals with generalizations, using empirical, statistical, and demographic methods or techniques. The idiographic approach typically involves the intense study of individuals (Allport, 1942, 1962). In suicidology, the intensive retrospective psychological study of a case (occurrence) is called a psychological autopsy. In this book we attempt to do both, the general and specific; it presents a literature review and an array of suicide cases; for example, some officers from the New York epidemic in 1934–1940, Lt. Michael Pigott, and Chief Thomas Moffatt; and a most unique case of homicide-suicide in police. We present verbatim, "Report to the London Police Service and London Community on the Deaths of David Lucio and Kelly Johnson" (Retrieved November 22, 2008 from the Web page of the London Police Service, www.police.london.ca). This book, we hope, meets the challenge at both a general (common) theoretical level and a forensic specific-case level of understanding. It will not meet all of the challenges, but it will in some ways.

As a crucial final point of introduction, there are of course views that theory should not play a role in understanding suicide; forensic study should only be at an individual-case level. (Will this answer all our questions?) We believe, however, that theory, explicit and implicit, plays a key role in understanding any behavior (it will allow us to wrap our heads around any case of suicide or homicide-suicide in police). Theory is the foundation of science (Kuhn, 1962) (and in sound police practice). Newton, Einstein, Ferri, Zilboorg, Shneidman, and all great scientists are great because they were theorists. It is only through theory, as Edwin Shneidman (1985) once noted, that we would sort out the booming buzzing mess of suicide and, we would add, suicide-homicide. Theory may well be in the eye of the beholder (Kuhn, 1962), but it is pivotal in understanding suicide among police and homicide followed by suicide, in police. This is as true for the forensic scientist as the officer. Theory, and associated technique of study, should be empirically based or evidence based—theory that can be and has been tested. It should not be armchair speculation. It should be subject to peer review and publication. It must have a standardized technique or method, and there has to be general acceptance. In fact, there is nothing as useful as good theory. We hope that it will help in understanding self-directed and other-directed lethal violence, and thus by application, in the prevention of such occurrences and in the healing in officers and community, once such a tragedy occurs, especially given the "blue walls" (barriers, stigma, dissembling) that have been documented before and after such events, since the very beginning of study of suicide among police in New York in the 1930s. And by implication, are there, thus, effective policies and procedures? What can be recommended?

There is, however, what is called the common forensic ecological fallacy; that is, making conclusions about an individual based solely on the general. To illustrate, suppose we take Dave, a law-enforcement officer of 22 years, and suppose his family background is marked with depression; his girlfriend rejected him; he is isolated; he received a demotion; his pain is unbearable; and he sees no escape from his malaise but suicide. Suppose that 70% of such officers, having a similar background, become suicidal. Does that mean that Dave has a 70% chance of killing himself? Echoing Allport, Murray, and Shneidman, the answer is no—not at all. Dave is a unique being. This is the very reason for this book.

Thus, to meet the challenge of outlining the state of the knowledge in suicide and homicide-suicide in police, we need to know both the nomothetic (general) and the idiographic (individual). We plan to present both, attempting to be mindful of the need of the officer on the street, the mental health provider, the administrator who must respond to the occurrence, and the survivors of the needless tragedies. It is our belief that by amalgamating the needs of a diverse audience, we can come closer to the challenge: who was officer Michael and why did he commit suicide? Or increasingly, why does an officer, Kelly, commit homicide-suicide?

Edwin Shneidman, a grandfather in the field and mentor, noted that the challenge in suicidology is the following: "We ought to know what we are talking about." It follows that we, both the officer and forensic specialist, need to know what we are investigating. Our study will be a difficult one; one must think outside the common blue or white frame (box). We cannot be cognitively constricted. We hope that this book helps, whether being suicidal; working with a fellow suicidal partner; administering to such an officer; providing mental health services to the officer and his or her police services; or surviving a loved one's homicide-suicide and working, after such a death, to assist in preventing further suicides and homicide-suicides in police. Thus, we are meeting the wish of almost all survivors of such tragedies, that something positive comes from the sting. We hope that it saves lives in police, their families, their fellow officers, and the community.

Antoon A. Leenaars

Acknowledgments

First and foremost, I need to make explicit my debt to Dr. Edwin Shneidman. Not only is his education central to my suicidological career, but also he first introduced me to the epidemic of police suicide. Under his birch tree at his Los Angeles home's back yard, we talked about the 93 suicides of the New York great suicide epidemic of the 1930s. Of note, there were five murder-suicides; this, we figured, would be well above expectations. Questions arose. Dr. Nancy Allen, his long-time friend, office partner at UCLA, and world expert on homicide, was often there with us at his home. We talked even more deeply about homicide-suicide. The works of Gregory Zilboorg, Paul Friedman, Donald West, and Marvin Wolfgang were consulted. We examined Dr. Allen's book, *Homicide* (1980); we specifically read pages 86–87 on murder-suicide. Dr. Shneidman even typed them out on his typewriter. (They can be found on pp. 102-103 of this book.) They were the most insightful conversations on the topic of homicide-suicide that I ever had. It was a stimulus for this book.

From the consultations, we concluded that homicide-suicide was suicide. We agreed on *a priori* concept: Suicide, and thus, homicide-suicide, is not only intrapsychic (existing or taking place within the mind or psyche), but also interpersonal, with a person, or, as Zilboorg had convincingly shown, an ideal. We then raised a most important question: on a continuum, when does a discrete individual event become a relationship one, from suicide pacts, ranging from co-equal involvement, such as lovers, to one of pressure and coercion, such as Arthur Koestler's and his wife, to unwilling victim and a perpetrator as in Dave Lucio and Kelly Johnson? (And today, I would add, to even mass murder-suicide of suicide bombers/terrorists, such as at 9/11.) In the 93 suicides of the New York police in the 1930s, could we have predicted the five homicide-suicides? Could we devise a blind experiment, using John Stuart Mill's method of difference, to predict and discriminate the five? Could we compare a sample of the 88 police suicides (non-homicides) with the five homicide-suicides? What empirically based knowledge would we thus learn? And why the police suicide and the higher rate of homicide-suicide in the New York police group? Could we investigate the survivors of the New York deaths? Could we do a psychological autopsy? (We knew of Jack Kamerman's work on the topic.) Could the homicides be sometimes victim precipitated? For all three of us, these questions and the answers were dynamic. Nancy Allen recommended a read of Sigmund Freud's *The Economic Problem of Masochism* (1974). (We would suggest not only that, but also Nancy's book, *Homicide*.) The excitement of those conversations at Ed Shneidman's home is hard to describe. Every word seemed like a new insight. Nancy later sent me her book, a collection of her favorite homicide books, old newspaper articles, her private notes on the topic of homicide and homicide-suicide. So did Ed. We discussed my many California homicide-suicide-attempt forensic cases, a number of very fertile, idiographic (individual) psychological autopsies (see Leenaars, 2002). One could want no better consultants. This book is a product of that education.

Of course, the adventure did not end there. Edwin Shneidman raised a challenge: "we ought to know what we are talking about." There is, it was obvious to all three of us, a need for this book. There are further acknowledgements needed, to meet that challenge, of course. This group included the following: Dr. Peter Collins (Ontario Provincial Police), Dr. Adriana Celser (Calgary Police Service), Detective David Gilmore (London Police Service), Prof. Jack Kamerman (Kean University, NJ), Myra Morant (Center for Suicide Prevention, Calgary, AB), and the survivors of police suicide. The survivors, through the psychological autopsies, taught me the individual (idiographic). We thank them for their cooperation, not only to understand the tragic events, but also for their input into the recommendations. The above group was most valuable.

We wish to acknowledge the writings of the following people: Gregory Zilboorg, Paul Friedman, John Violanti, Robert Loo, and Steven Stack. We borrow here and there verbatim from their work on the topic. There are many other authors, too many to list (the references give us a state of the knowledge). Much of our recommendations are common in police service. We fully acknowledge the following services that unquestionably assisted us in our book and recommendations: Ontario Provincial Police (OPP); Calgary Police Service (CPS); London Police Service (LPS); Centre for Suicide Prevention (CSP), Calgary, AB; Federal Bureau of Investigation (FBI, their book, *Suicide and Law Enforcement* is a must read); and the International Association of Chiefs of Police. There are many more individuals and services. Dank U (Dutch for thank you, but a little more).

The support of my family is always appreciated, especially of Brian Egan, my son-in-law and Officer of Border Security Services, Canada. Brian; my wife, Susanne; and my daughter, Lindsey, read the text; so did Peter Collins and Dave Gilmore. I needed a police input to the volume if it was going to be of value to police officers, of course. Their various suggestions improved the book.

I want to thank Dale Lund; we are also appreciative of the two anonymous reviewers, and the excellent editorial staff at Baywood; I first purposely sent them this volume because of their comprehensive list on both topics of suicide and police.

Appreciation is acknowledged to all the following with permission, if needed under Copyright Act, to reproduce materials that appear in this volume.

Excerpts from N. Allen, (1980). *Homicide*. New York: Human Sciences Press. Within "fair use" of copyrighted material.

Excerpts from B. Danto, (1978). Police suicide. *Police Stress, 1,* 32–40. Within "fair use" of copyrighted material.

Excerpts from P. Friedman, (1967a). Suicide among police: A study of 93 suicides among New York policemen, 1934–1940. In E. Shneidman (Ed.), *Essays in self-destruction* (pp. 415–449). New York: Jason Aronson, Inc. (By permission of Dr. Edwin S. Shneidman).

Excerpts from J. Kamerman, (1993). The illegacy of suicide. In A. Leenaars (Ed.), *Suicidology: Essays in honor of Edwin S. Shneidman* (pp. 346–355). Northvale, NJ: Jason Aronson, Inc. (By permission of the Rowan & Littlefield Publishing Group).

Excerpts from R. Loo, (1986). Suicide among police in a federal force. *Suicide & Life-Threatening Behavior, 16,* 379–385. Within "fair use" of copyrighted material.

Excerpts from R. Loo, (2001). Effective postvention for police suicide. *The Australian Journal of Disaster & Trauma Studies,* 2001–2002. Retrieved 2001, from http://www.massey.ac.nz/~trauma1 (By permission of Prof. Douglas Paton, Editor, The Australian J. of Disaster & Trauma Studies).

Report from A. Leenaars, P. Collins, and D. Sinclair, (May 20, 2008). Report to the London Police Service and London Community on the Deaths of David Lucio and Kelly Johnson. In public domain.

Excerpts from E. Pam, (2001). Police homicide-suicide in relation to domestic violence. In D. Sheehan & J. Warren (Eds.), *Suicide and law enforcement* (pp. 357–363). Washington, DC: FBI. In public domain.

Excerpts from W. Powers, (1999). Confidentiality and counselling. *Personnel files, Chicago Police Department, 1–2,* 1. In public domain.

Excerpts from E. Shneidman, (1977). The psychological autopsy. In L. Gottshalk (Ed.), *Guide to investigation and reporting of drug abuse deaths.* U. S. Government Printing Office, Washington, DC: US DHEW. In public domain.

Excerpts from S. Stack, (1997). Homicide followed by suicide: An analysis of Chicago data. *Criminology, 35,* 435–453. (By permission of Dr. Steven Stack and American Society of Criminology).

Excerpts from J. Violanti, (2001). Police suicide: Current perspectives and future considerations. In D. Sheehan & J. Warren (Eds.), *Suicide and law enforcement* (pp. 437–446). Washington, DC: FBI. In public domain.

Excerpts from J. Violanti, (2007). Homicide-suicide in police families: Aggression full circle. *International Journal of Emergency Mental Health, 9,* 97–104. (By permission of Chevron Publishing Co.).

OTHELLO

Act 5, Scene II

Act 5, Scene II. *A bedchamber in the castle:* Desdemona *in bed asleep; a light burning*

Enter Othello.

Oth. It is the cause, it is the cause, my soul –
Let me not name it to you, you chaste stars! –
It is the cause. Yet I'll not shed her blood;
Nor scar that whiter skin of hers than snow,
And smooth as monumental alabaster.
Yet she must die, else she'll betray more men.
Put out the light, and then put out the light.
If I quench thee, thou flaming minister,
I can again thy former light restore.
Should I repent me; but once put out thy light,
Thou cunning'st pattern of excelling nature,
I know not where is that Promethean heat
That can thy light relume. When I have pluck'd
the rose
I cannot give it vital growth again,
It must needs wither. I'll smell it on the tree.
Kissing her.
Ah, balmy breath, that dost almost persuade
Justice to break her sword! One more, one more.
Be thus when thou art dead, and I will kill thee,
And love thee after. One more, and this the last;
So sweet was ne'er so fatal. I must weep,
But they are cruel tears. This sorrow's heavenly;
It strikes where it doth love. She wakes.
Des. Who's there? Othello?
Oth. Ay, Desdemona.
Des. Will you come to bed, my lord?

Oth. Have you pray'd to-night, Desdemona?
Des. Ay, my lord.
Oth. If you think yourself of any crime
Unreconciled as yet to Heaven and grace,
Solicit for it straight.
Des. Alas, my lord, what do you mean by that?
Oth. Well, do it, and be brief; I will walk by.
I would not kill thy unprepared spirit;
No, heaven forfend! I would not kill thy soul.
Des. Talk you of killing?
Oth. Ay, I do.
Des. Then Heaven
Have mercy on me!
Oth. Amen, with all my heart!
Des. If you say so, I hope you will not kill me.
Oth. Hum!
Des. And yet I fear you; for you are fatal then
When your eyes roll so. Why I should fear I
know not,
Since guiltiness I know not; but yet I feel I fear.
Oth. Think on thy sins.
Des. They are loves I bear to you.
Oth. Ay, and for that thou diest.
Des. That death's unnatural that kills for loving.
Alas, why gnaw you so your nether lip?
Some bloody passion shakes your very frame.
These are portents; but yet I hope, I hope,
They do not point on me.
Oth. Peace, and be still!
Des. I will so. What's the matter?
Oth. That handkerchief which I so loved and
Gave thee
Thou gavest to Cassio.
Des. No, by my life and soul!
Send for the man, and ask him.
Oth. Sweet soul, take heed,
Take heed of perjury; thou art on thy death-bed.
Des. Ay, but not yet to die.
Oth. Yes, presently;
Therefore confess thee freely of thy sin;
For to deny each article with oath

Cannot remove nor choke the strong conception
That I do groan withal. Thou art to die.
Des. Then Lord have mercy on me!
Oth. I say, amen.
Des. And have you mercy too! I never did
Offend you in my life; never loved Cassio
But with much general warranty of heaven
As I might love; I never gave him token.
Oth. By heaven, I saw my handkerchief in's
hand.
O perjured woman! thou dost stone my heart,
And makest me call what I intend to do
A murder, which I thought a sacrifice.
I saw the handkerchief.
Des. He found it then;
I never gave it him. Send for him hither;
Let him confess a truth.
Oth. He hath confess'd.
Des. What, my lord?
Oth. That he hath used thee.
Des. How? unlawfully?
Oth. Ay.
Des. He will not say so.
Oth. No, his mouth is stopp'ed;
Honest Iago hath ta'en order for't.
Des. O! my fear interprets. What, is he dead?
Oth. Had all his hairs been lives, my great re-
venge
Had stomach for them all.
Des. Alas! He is betray'd and I undone.
Oth. Out, strumpet! weep'st thou for him to my
face?
Des. O, banish me, my lord, but kill me not!
Oth. Down, strumpet!
Des. Kill me to-morrow; let me live to-night!
Oth. Nay, if you strive-
Des. But half an hour!
Oth. Being done, there is no pause.
Des. But while I say one prayer!
Oth. It is too late
He stifles her.

After killing Desdemona, his wife, and stating, "My wife! my wife! what wife? I have no wife. O, insupportable! O heavy hour!" and stabbing himself, Othello claims:

Oth. Soft you; a word or two before you go.
I have done the state some service, and they know't.
No more of that. I pray you, in your letters,
When you shall these unlucky deeds relate,
Speak of me as I am; nothing extenuate,
Nor set down auth in malice. Then must you
Speak
Of one that loved not wisely but too well;
Of one not easily jealous, but being wrought
Perplex'd in the extreme; of one whose hand,
Like the base Indian, threw a pearl away
Richer than all his tribe; of one whose subdued
eyes,
Albeit unused to the melting mood,
Drop tears as fast as the Arabian trees
Their medicinal gum. Set you down this,
And say besides, that in Aleppo once,
Where a malignant and turban'd Turk
Beat a Venetian and traduced the state,
I took by the throat the circumcised dog,
And smote him, thus. [*Stabs himself.*]
Lod. O bloody period!
Gra. All that's spoke is marr'd.
Oth. I kiss'd thee ere I kill'd thee. No way but
This.
Killing myself, to die upon a kiss.
[*Falls on the bed and dies.*]

Othello,
Act 5, Scene II
William Shakespeare

CHAPTER 1

Suicide

Shakespeare said it so well hundreds of years ago. He knew suicide. There are some 52 suicides in his writings. Moreover, there is the most famous forensic study, *Othello*, the most documented homicide-suicide in history. Edwin Shneidman's contributions are no different; he is a grandfather of forensic suicidology—he invented, named, and had others invest in the field. He developed such concepts as psychological autopsy, subintentional death, and postvention. He defined the term, suicide, as follows:

> Currently in the Western world, suicide is a conscious act of self-induced annihilation, best understood as a multidimensional malaise in a needful individual who defines an issue for which suicide is perceived as the best solution.

One should reflect on each word and the *Gestalt* for the individual case and the general (idiographic and nomothetic approaches). Of course, there are many more important theorists; we will meet them in this chapter. There are leading suicidologists to guide us, beyond Shneidman. They are Alfred Adler, Ludwig Binswanger, Sigmund Freud, Carl Jung, George Kelly, Karl Menninger, Henry Murray, Harry Stack Sullivan, and Gregory Zilboorg. We learn that not only Shakespeare and Shneidman, but all great forensic theorists on suicide believe that although suicide is more, insofar as it is psychology, it stems from the person's unbearable psychological pain, from personal anguish, perturbation, and *pain*. Given this central idea, all the rest in this chapter is explication of the details.

Shneidman thought that, "We need to know what we are talking about." We agree. We believe that we will investigate (and know) major crime scenes, such as suicide, more effectively only when we develop evidence-based (or fact-based) understanding of suicide, whether the general or the unique case in police. (Are they that different?) Indeed, we believe that in the study of forensic (police) issues like suicide, there is a natural progression from conceptualization to understanding, and then to applied practice, whether on the street, the crime scene, or the office of the Psychological Services Section of a police department. This section serves like an introductory course to our topic (we can call it Suicidology Among Police, 101). It consists of a number of sections: definition of suicide; intentional,

http://dx.doi.org/10.2190/SHSC1

subintentional and unintentional; suicide facts and myths; attempted suicide; forensic observations; and behavioral clues. We will read some of the most personal documents written—the suicide note. After, we will move to the evaluation of suicide risk, a most difficult of tasks, sometimes lethal, if one miscalculates the risk (such as "suicide by cop").

The concept of assessment is preferable to that of diagnosis; with police, we do not need only a diagnostic approach (one will be called "Doc Nuts"). There is no one clue, or sign, or evidence. Equally, the search for a singular tool for evidence collection or question is a chimera, a myth. This section reflects today's science of suicide risk assessment, a disappointing one. It is difficult, and may well be the most difficult that a police officer, clinician, and forensic scientist face. Thus, we will address the question, how do we predict suicide in police? After a free association on the topic of sex differences, we finally present a theory of suicide, the foundation of our forensic work. We learn some commonalities. These are the "threads" of behavior that run through the suicidal person's life history. We can learn much. There is evidence. There are, in fact, consistent threads in every case of police suicide. It is a survey or outline of suicide. It gives a conspectus: to give a summary of the psychological aspects of suicide in terms of its common and ubiquitous characteristics, with a most rare cross-cultural application.

Suicide is a psychological drama on an interpersonal stage; this is so for police. Suicide can be clinically understood from at least, the following templates or commonalities of the intrapsychic (within the mind) factors: unbearable psychological pain, cognitive constriction (or narrow thinking), indirect expressions (or unconscious processes), emotional disturbances (or psychopathology), and a feeling of being vulnerable (ego). The common interpersonal factors are problematic relationships, rejection-aggression, and a wish to escape. These elements have utility in understanding suicide, as well as predicting and preventing the same. The evidence for the theory is presented. Not only due to the high incidence of police suicide, but also to the keen interest in forensic suicidology, a note on cognitive style and dissembling are presented, the latter being so figural in police. The following question is asked: "How is it that some officers who are on the verge of suicide—and some before murder—can hide or mask their secretly held intentions?" This is called masking or dissembling. (No officer should underestimate this concept.)

Shneidman, among others such as Harry Murray, have explicitly supported the intensive study of a unique case, what Shneidman called a *psychological autopsy*. Murray's most important (and his proudest) psychological case (specific) investigation was of the personality of Adolf Hitler; he was an officer with the Office of the Strategic Services (OSS), an intelligence agency of the U.S. federal government. Murray predicted the violence and murders, followed by Hitler's suicide, a homicide(s)-suicide. We present the unique case of Vince Foster Jr., former-President Bill Clinton's deputy White House council, who shot himself. The specific (unique) case shows us more of the suicidal mind (and we will meet many such officers). Likewise, on a day-to-day basis, we, officers and forensic specialists, are interested in the unique officer. Our practical question is, How do we assess that officer's suicide risk? Is he or she suicidal? To what extent was the homicide-suicide predictable and preventable? Murray predicted that Hitler would "die, dragging all of Europe with him into the abyss." Could it have been prevented? Can an officer's suicide be predicted or prevented? What safeguards could be in place to reduce the risk of future incidents? These too are aims of this somewhat long chapter and the whole volume: to save lives.

* * * * * *

INTRODUCTION

Suicide is a multidimensional event (Leenaars, 1993a, 1999a, 2004; Shneidman, 1973, 1985; Zilboorg, 1937). Suicide and suicidal behavior are multifaceted events. There are biological, psychological, intrapsychic, interpersonal, sociological, cultural, and philosophical elements in the event. Thus, suicide and suicidal behavior cannot be reduced to a single factor. This complexity of causation indicates the necessity of a parallel complexity of knowledge. Indeed, because suicide is a multifaceted problem, it needs to be understood on several different levels at once. This is equally true of homicide (Allen, 1980) and what presents to us too often, homicide-suicide. We will explore these topics, but we will first discuss suicide in some detail. One, unequivocally, has to know suicide to understand a suicidal or suicidal-homicidal officer.

Most frequently, people identify external causes (e.g., ill health, being abandoned by a lover, a demotion) as to why the person killed himself. This view is too simplistic, although often the suicidal person holds that perspective. This is not to suggest that a recent traumatic event (e.g., a divorce, loss of a parent) cannot be identified in many suicides. However, although there are always situational aspects in every suicidal act, they are only one aspect of the complexity, which we hope to demonstrate in this book.

Suicide is a multidimensional malaise (Shneidman, 1985). Suicide is not a sin. Suicide is not a crime. (It has been decriminalized in most of the world.) Suicide, rather, is a state of being, a human malaise. Malaise, according to the *Oxford English Dictionary* (OED) is "a condition of . . . discomfort . . . a feeling of uneasiness." Malaise is PAIN. It is the deepest anguish (angst). There are biological, psychological, intrapsychic, logical, conscious and unconscious, interpersonal, sociological, cultural, and philosophical/existential elements in the suicidal pain, to name a few.

Any element of the malaise is a legitimate avenue to understanding suicide. Studies of serotonin have a place. Studies of police culture have a place. Studies of the effect of gun control have a place. In fact, we oppose any reductionistic model in understating suicide. Suicide is a multifaceted event and is open to study by multiple disciplines; herein we offer a forensic psychological/psychiatric perspective. Let us begin with Shneidman's (1985) arboreal image to understand suicide. He wrote:

> An individual's biochemical states, for instance, are the roots. An individual's method of suicide, the contents of the suicide note, the calculated effects on the survivors and so on, are the branching limbs, the flawed fruit, and the camouflaging leaves. But the psychological component, the problem solving choice, the best solution of the perceived problem, is the main "trunk." (pp. 202–203)

From a psychological point of view, we would like to offer a few observations on the question, "why?"

DEFINITION OF SUICIDE

Understanding begins with definition. Briefly defined, suicide is the human act of self-inflicted, self-intentioned cessation (Shneidman, 1973). Suicide is not a disease (although there are many who think so); it is not a biological anomaly (although biological factors may play a role in some suicides); it is not an immorality (although it has often been treated as such); and it is not a crime in the United States, Canada, and most countries around the world (although it was for centuries).

Suicide may today be defined differently depending on the purpose of the definition—medical, legal, administrative, and so on. In the United States and Canada (and most of the countries reporting to the World Health Organization [WHO]), suicide is defined (by a medical examiner or coroner) as one of the four possible modes of death. An acronym for the four modes of death is NASH: natural, accidental, suicidal, and homicidal. This fourfold classification of all deaths has its problems. The major deficiency is that it treats the human being in a Cartesian fashion, namely as a biological machine, rather than appropriately treating her as a motivated, intentional, biopsychosocial organism; that is, it obscures the individual's intentions in relation to her own cessation and, further, completely neglects the contemporary concepts of psychodynamic psychology regarding intention, including unconscious motivation.

The topic of the definition of suicide was the focus of an entire book by Shneidman (1985). *Definition of Suicide* can be seen as a necessary step to more effective understanding and prevention of suicide. In the book, Shneidman (1985) argued that we desperately need a clarification of the definitions of suicide— definitions that can be applied to needful persons. He defined suicide as:

> Currently in the Western world, suicide is a conscious act of self-induced annihilation, best understood as a multidimensional malaise in a needful individual who defines an issue for which the suicide is perceived as the best solution. (p. 203)

We will be using Shneidman's definition here.

The two giants in the field of suicidal theorizing at the turn of the 20th century were Emile Durkheim and Sigmund Freud. Durkheim, in *Suicide* (1897/1951), focused on society's inimical effects on the individual, while Freud, eschewing the notions of either sin or crime, gave suicide back to intentional man, but put the locus of action in man's unconscious. Since around 1900, a host of psychological theories aside from Freud's have focused on the individual; for example, those of Alfred Adler, Ludwig Binswanger, Carl G. Jung, George Kelly, Karl Menninger, Henry A. Murray, Edwin Shneidman, Harry Stack Sullivan, and Gregory Zilboorg, to name some of the best known (Leenaars, 1988). These suicidologists have given us a rich history to understand suicide; thus, we will use these suicidologists' theories to understand suicide in police and homicide-suicide in police.

INTENTIONAL, SUBINTENTIONAL, AND UNINTENTIONAL

Freud (1901/1974), Shneidman (1963), Murray (1967), and others have speculated that beyond intentional suicides, there is a vast array of subintentional inimical behaviors. The very lifestyle of some police officers, for example, seems to truncate and demean their life, so that they are as good as dead. In 1901, Freud stated,

> It is well known that in the severe cases of psychoneurosis instances of self injury are occasionally found as symptoms and that in such cases suicide can never be ruled out as a possible outcome of the physical conflict . . . many apparently accidental injuries that happen to such patients are really instances of self-injury. (pp. 178–179)

Freud further notes that such self-destruction is not rare. Often alcoholism, drug addiction, mismanagement of service guns, high-speed car chases, and masochistic behavior can be seen in this light (Farberow, 1980; Murphy, 1992). We, in this volume, will explore the many faces of suicide.

A related concept is "subintentioned death" (Shneidman, 1963). This concept asserts that there are many deaths that are neither clearly suicidal nor clearly accidental or natural. These are deaths in which the decedent played some covert or unconscious role in "permitting" his or her death to occur, either "accidentally" or by "inviting" homicide, or by unconsciously disregarding what could be a life-extending medical regimen, and thus dying sooner than "necessary." Freud (1901) speculated,

> Anyone who believes in the occurrence of half-intentional self-injury—if I may use a clumsy expression—will be prepared also to assume that in addition to consciously intentional suicide there is such a thing as half-intentional self-destruction (self-destruction with an unconscious intention), capable of making skilful use of a threat of life and of disguising it as a chance mishap. (pp. 180–181)

An important aspect of the issue at hand is that suicide is an intentional act. As Litman (1984) noted,

> The concept, which defines a death as suicide rather than an accident, is intention. For example, we assume that when a man shoots himself in the head with a gun, he intended to die. Therefore the death was a suicide. However, if in fact, he intended to survive, for example, if he thought the gun was not loaded, the death was accidental. (p. 88)

Litman (1984) provides some striking insights on the topic. The case of the actor Freddie Prinze, is an example in point, he stated. Freddie Prinze shot himself in the head one night with his manager present. Mr. Prinze had called several people, stating, "I'm going to do it." He wrote a note in which he stated, "No one is responsible." The question here was, even if he left a note, was the death intentional? A few other facts were critical, according to Litman (1984). Freddie Prinze was a drug user and had used drugs that night, and he often played with guns, often mimicking shooting himself. The decision, at least for insurance purposes, in that case was that he did not intend to kill himself. To conclude, the question to determine the mode of death as a suicide is: did the person intentionally kill himself?

Therefore, we are well advised to keep the concept of intentional, subintentional, and unintentional in mind, especially in forensic cases (Litman, 1988).

SUICIDE FACTS AND MYTHS

Lore about suicide contains a large number of interesting and esoteric items. People in general are not only perplexed and bewildered by self-destructive behavior, but they also believe a number of misconceptions of suicide. Here are some common fables and facts about suicide, formulated by Shneidman around 1952 and incorporated into a number of publications (e.g., Shneidman & Mandelkorn, 1967):

1. Fable: People who talk about suicide don't commit suicide.
   Fact: Of any 10 persons, who kill themselves, 8 have given definite warnings of their suicidal intentions.
2. Fable: Suicide happens without warning.
   Fact: Studies reveal that the suicidal person gives many clues and warnings regarding suicidal intentions.
3. Fable: Suicidal people are fully intent on dying.
   Fact: Most suicidal people are undecided about living or dying, and they "gamble with death," leaving it to others to save them. Almost no one commits suicide without letting others know how they are feeling.

4. Fable: Once a person is suicidal he or she is suicidal forever.
   Fact: Individuals who wish to kill themselves are suicidal only for a limited period of time.
5. Fable: Improvement following a suicidal crisis means that the suicidal risk is over.
   Fact: Most suicides occur within about three months following the beginning of "improvement," when the individual has the energy to put his morbid thoughts and feelings into effect.
6. Fable: Suicide strikes much more often among the rich—or, conversely, it occurs most exclusively among the poor.
   Fact: Suicide is neither the rich person's disease nor the poor person's curse. Suicide is very "democratic" and is represented proportionately among all levels of society.
7. Fable: All suicidal individuals are mentally ill, and suicide always is the act of a psychotic person.
   Fact: Studies of hundreds of genuine suicide notes indicate that although the suicidal person is extremely unhappy, he is not necessarily mentally ill.

ATTEMPTED SUICIDE

A previous attempt is one of the best clues to future attempts (Beck, Kovacs, & Weissman, 1975). However, not all previous attempters go on to attempt again (or kill themselves; about 15% do so versus 1.5% for the general population [Leenaars & Lester, 1994a; Lester, 1992a]). Although it is obvious that one has to attempt suicide in order to commit it, it is equally clear that the event of attempting suicide does not always have death (cessation) as its objective. It is acknowledged that often the goal of attempted suicide (such as cutting oneself or ingesting large amounts of alcohol) is to change one's life (or to change the behavior of the significant others around one) rather than to end it (Shneidman, 1985). However, we wish to stress, as have others (e.g., Stengel, 1964), that it is useful to think of the "attempter," sometimes referred to as the parasuicide, and the "completer," as two sets of overlapping populations:

1. a group of those who attempt suicide, a few of whom go on to commit it; and
2. a group of those who commit suicide, many of whom previously attempted it. A great deal has to do with *perturbation* and *lethality* associated with the event.

Perturbation refers to how upset (disturbed, agitated, sane-insane) the individual is—rated as low-medium-high (or alternatively on a 1 to 9 scale)—and may be measured by various means (e.g., self-reports, biological markers, psychological tests, observations). Lethality is roughly synonymous with the "deathfulness" of the act and is an important dimension in understanding any potentially suicidal individual. Lethality can be rated as low-moderate-high (or alternatively on a 1 to 9 scale). An example for measuring lethality is the following assessment item, derived from Shneidman (1967): "During the last 24 hours, I felt the chances of my actually killing myself (committing suicide and ending my life) were: absent, very low, low-medium, fifty-fifty, high medium, very high, extra high (came very close to actually killing myself)." A critical distinction in suicide (and often, for that matter, homicide) is that lethality—not perturbation—kills. All sorts of people are highly perturbed but are not suicidal. The ratio between suicide attempts and completions is about 4 to 1 to about 8 to 1—one committed suicide for every four to eight attempts; however, in young people, some reports have the ratio at 50 to 1, even 100 to 1. The ratio, in fact, appears to vary a lot between nations and across risk groups, sex, age, and so on.

FORENSIC OBSERVATIONS

This section consists of six parts, sometimes called contextual clues, focused on clarifying suicide, biological roots, brain dysfunctions, physical disabilities and illness, depression, specific precipitating events, and the family system.

Biological Roots

"No brain, no mind" is one of Henry Murray's reminders to his student Edwin Shneidman (Shneidman, 2001). Dr. Shneidman's position is best presented in his 1985 book, *Definition of Suicide*. Therein, he states his principles (see his Chapter V, "A formal definition, with explication"). He writes,

> Suicide is a multifaceted event and that biological, cultural, sociological, interpersonal, intrapsychic, logical, conscious and unconscious, and philosophical elements are present, in various degrees, in each suicidal event. (p. 202)

Stoff and Mann's (1997) edited volume begins to outline the current understanding of the neurobiology of suicide. On a critical note, however, one could see Stoff and Mann's view as being too reductionistic. They reduce suicide to only biological roots. Stoff and Mann write,

> Efforts aimed at identifying the potentially suicidal individual using demographic, social developmental and psychological factors offer too weak a prediction to be of substantial clinical utility. It is believed that the biological perspective, which has grown out of the expanding research on the biological basis of mood disorders, is a predominant approach to suicide research. It can assist in the investigation of risk factors that predispose a person to suicidal behavior and that increase understanding of etiology, treatment, and ultimately, prevention. (p. 1)

Utilizing only this view will lead us astray. (A person is not simply a biological anomaly.) Once more, suicide is complex, more complex than most people are aware. It is not only the suicidal brain. It is not only the suicidal mind.

The classical study in suicidology of the biological roots was by Asberg, Traskman, and Thorien (1976). They identified 5-H1 AA in cerebrospinal fluid as a biochemical marker in some suicides. This study marked the beginning of empirical biological suicidology. Yet although the Asberg study is now over 30 years old, there is relatively little well-documented, verified knowledge regarding the neurobiology of suicide today (Hawton & van Heeringen, 2000).

Despite the state of the knowledge, suicide must be seen as a biological event (and much more). Possible markers, isolated to date, include urinary 17-hydroxycorticosteroids (17-OHCS); cortisol in plasma and cerebrospinal fluid; cerebrospinal fluid 5-hydroxyindoleacetic acid; tritiated imipramine binding; 3-methoxy-4-hydroxyphenylglycol and homovanillic acid; urinary norepinephrine/epinephrine ratio; and thyroid-stimulating hormone response to thyrotropin-releasing hormone. Slaby (1992) and others (e.g., Maltsberger, 2002) are optimistic about our biological understanding of suicide in the future, especially in the relation of suicide to affective disorders (e.g., manic-depressive disorder) and their neurobiological correlates. At least, in some suicides, biological correlates may be strikingly relevant.

Brain Dysfunction and Learning Disabilities

The importance of brain dysfunction and its relation to cognitive deficits, learning disabilities, aggression (violence) regulation, and other abilities, are well documented. The relation of brain dysfunction and socioemotional problems in people is, however, a more neglected topic in the literature. Not only does a cognitive disorder (or learning disability or even Alzheimer's) render a person at-risk for socioemotional problems including suicide, but also there are particular subtypes of impairments/disabilities that may result in different levels of risk. Rourke and Fisk (1981) have documented that different patterns of cerebral dysfunction and their resulting disability(ies) render a person at-risk for different types of socioemotional disturbances. They report three major subgroups: The first group has a right-brain dysfunction. These people are prone to learning problems with nonverbal, visual information. They may show the following socioemotional problems: not paying attention to visual objects including other people (such as in a suicide by cop situation); rarely expressing emotions appropriately in their facial expressions; having a voice that can be expressionless; being very talkative; talking to self; having flow problems in their speech; and being awkward socially. The second group has a left-brain dysfunction. These people are prone to learning problems with verbal information. They may show the following socioemotional problems: rarely initiating conversations (even in the station's locker room); having problems paying attention, for example, in conversation; being brief and often concrete in their remarks; often stating "I don't know" to questions; and some are very impulsive, not thinking before they act. The third group has both left- and right-brain dysfunction and exhibit a conglomerate of symptoms.

Other more specific cerebral deficits render people at risk for other specific problems such as planning, sequencing social events, and so on; sometimes there are problems in executive functioning (such as mood regulation, thinking before acting, and so on). Attention deficit/hyperactivity disorder (ADHD), in all its subtypes, is an example. There are officers, for example, with ADHD, some with very high IQs. There are diverse brain dysfunctions, some chronic, while some are acute. The acute may be due to strokes or to recovery after being hit with a bullet in the head such as in a gang shootout situation (or in self-inflicted shooting). There are many work-related injuries or other risk factors in some police officers. Although further empirical studies need to be conducted in the neuropsychology of suicides, these observations clearly warrant attention. Indeed, Rourke, Young, and Leenaars (1989) have shown that one possible adolescent and adult outcome of childhood brain (central processing) deficiencies is suicidal behavior as well as other socioemotional problems, such as depression. They suggested that it is especially the first pattern associated with right-brain dysfunction that predisposes those afflicted to adolescent and adult suicide risk. This can all be true in acute cases of brain trauma in officers. The brain is so critical in risk.

Physical Disabilities and Illness

We would be remiss if we did not at least note the importance of physical problems in suicidal behavior in some people (Barraclough, 1986; Marzuk, 1994; Stenger & Stenger, 2000), and this is especially true in policing, given the large number of work-related injuries. Physical illness interacts with an individual's emotional functioning; indeed, some illnesses directly affect one's emotions. Empirical study regarding illness and suicide is urgently needed: currently research suggests that some physical illnesses are associated with suicidal behavior, including anorexia, bulimia, diabetes, epilepsy, traumatic brain injury (as we discussed above) and muscular dystrophia (Barraclough, 1986). Menstruation dysfunction and suicide are highly correlated (Dogra et al., 2007). Some individuals with physical disabilities who are at risk are those with limb amputations or spinal injuries resulting in quadriplegia. Individuals with terminal illness such as AIDS appear also to be at high risk (Marzuk, 1989). However, it is important to realize that not all such people are suicidal and that research is needed to substantiate these views.

Depression

It was once believed that all suicidal people were depressed, but this is a myth. The fact is that not all suicidal people are depressed, and that not all depressed people are suicidal. Depression and suicide are not equivalent. Yet Lester (1992a) has noted that depression distinguishes many suicidal people from nonsuicidal groups. Depression can be noted in mood and behavior (ranging from feeling dejected and hesitancy in social contacts, to isolation and serious disturbance of appetite and sleep), verbal expression (ranging from talks about being disappointed, excluded, blamed, etc., to talk of suicide, being killed, abandoned, helpless), and fantasy (ranging from feeling disappointed, excluded, mistreated, etc., to suicide, mutilation, loss of a significant person) (Pfeffer, 1986). Behaviors such as excessive aggressiveness, change in work performance, and expressions of somatic complaints or loss of energy have all been associated with depression. However, not all depression is overt; some may be masked or guarded. Some people exhibit what has been termed masked depression. They dissemble. Anorexia, promiscuity, and alcohol abuse, for example, have been associated with depression, but also many other emotional disturbances or behaviors, too many to list. It is important to remember, however, that depression does not equal suicide in a simple one to one fashion. Most suicides experience unbearable pain, but not necessarily depression (Shneidman, 1985). The unbearable emotion might be hostility, anxiety, despair, shame, guilt, dependency, hopelessness, or helplessness. What is critical is that the emotion—pain—is unbearable. Unendurable psychological pain is the common stimulus in suicide (Shneidman, 1985), not depression alone.

Specific Environmental Precipitating Events

A current popular formulation regarding suicide is that suicide is simply due to an external event; for example, a rejection by a lover; the loss of a gun of a police officer; an investigation into a lethal order of misusing a Taser on an emotionally disturbed person, whatever. Of course, like all people, precipitating events (e.g., abuse of alcohol, sexual deviance, being bullied by supervisors, death of parent, divorce, a demotion) do occur in the suicides of police. That event is often difficult to discern. We are here reminded of a clinical example: A 16-year veteran police officer was found dead in his car, having died of carbon monoxide poisoning. People were perplexed: "Why did this person from an upper-middle-class family kill himself?" The parents found out that his girlfriend rejected him the day of his suicide. That was the reason: when a person gets rejected and is so in love, he may kill himself. A few friends and his Sergeant at the police service knew that he had been having problems at work and was facing a demotion. That was the reason. A few others knew that his father was an alcoholic and abusive in his childhood. That was the reason. His physician knew that he had been depressed, had not taking his prescribed medication, and had been recently upset about that ("I'll be in the nut house next.") She knew the real reason. And others knew . . . (What do you know about the officer who died by suicide?)

Shneidman (1985) has noted that the common consistency in suicide is not the precipitating event, but lifelong coping patterns. There are enduring characteristics, sometimes a personality disorder. People who kill themselves experience a steady toll of threat, stress, failure, challenge, and loss that gradually undermine their adjustment process. Suicide has a history.

There are, of course, many threats, stresses, and so on in the suicidal person's mind. One further stimulus that has frequently been identified as a possible precipitating event is the death of a well-known, much publicized suicide. The discussion raises the issues of the contagion (copycat) effect. Some years ago in Japan, for example, an 18-year-old pop idol, Yukiko Okada, after a fight with her lover, leaped to her death from the building that housed her recording company in Tokyo. In the 17 days following her suicide, the suicide toll reached 33 people. Phillips (1974, 1986) has documented the fact that such cluster suicides do occur in adults, unequivocally. Suicide clusters have, in fact, been reported in Japan, North America, and across the world. Suicide clusters have also been reported in police services. Aside from clustering, the impact of suggestion is also seen in the effect of media reporting of suicide. Most recently, it has been noted that there may be particular characteristics of contagion suicides (Brent, 1992; Martin, 1998). This raises a question: Did the officer's homicide-suicide have an impact on vulnerable people? Was there a contagion? Only a research study, analyzing about 2 to 6 years before/after of all area suicides, homicides, homicide-suicide(s) can answer this question, empirically, but one should keep contagion in mind after the death of an officer.

Family Background

A review of the literature (e.g., Berman & Jobes, 1991; Leenaars & Wenckstern, 1991; Maris, 1981; Pfeffer, 1986; Richman, 1991, 1993; Toolan, 1981) suggests that the family system and its functioning is a central factor associated with suicide and suicidal behavior, although by no means do all families show these characteristics—some, none at all. Nevertheless, a few common observations of families are here provided:

1. There is, at times, a lack of generational boundaries in suicidal families. There is an insufficient separation of the parent from his family of origin. For example, a parent may take over the role of selecting and even being reinforcing of a career, such as being a law enforcement officer, well within adulthood.
2. The family system is often inflexible. Any change is seen as a threat to the survival of the family. Denial, secretiveness, dissembling, and especially a lack of communication characterize the family's interactions. This is especially so in the suicides of police, but also for more reasons than the familial ones. Denial is often a lethal event.

3. At times there is a symbiotic parent-child relationship. A parent, usually the mother, is too attached to the child, even the adult child. Not only is such a relation disturbing, but the parent also does not provide the emotional protection and support that a parent usually provides intuitively to a person as she grows. Additionally, it has been noted repeatedly that if such a parent dies, the person may kill herself to be magically reunited with that same parent.
4. Long-term disorganization (malfunctioning) has been noted in these families; for example, mother's or father's control, divorce, domestic violence, alcoholism, or mental illness. In women, there is a very high rate of incest, sexual abuse, or such compared with the general population.

These observations raise further questions: Are the familial/interpersonal factors identified due to psychopathology, not suicide risk per se? What are the familial risk factors of officers? Protective factors?

BEHAVIORAL CLUES

In understanding suicide, we need to be aware of behaviors that are potentially predictive of suicide. However, there is no single definitive predictive behavior. The two concepts, which have already been discussed, that may be helpful here are lethality and perturbation. The clues below are applicable to all age groups, although the mode of expression may differ depending on age and numerous other factors. Loo (2001), Miller (2005), and Violanti (2001) present excellent papers on clues to suicide in police officers; we below, here and there, add our insights.

Previous Attempts

Although it is obvious that one has to attempt suicide in order to commit it, it is equally clear that the event of attempting suicide need not have death as its objective. As noted earlier, it is useful to think of overlapping populations:

1. a group of those who attempt suicide, a few of whom go on to commit it; and
2. a group of those who commit suicide, many of whom previously attempted it.

A previous attempt is a good clue to future attempts, especially if no assistance is obtained after the first attempt. However, not all previous attempters go on to attempt again (or kill themselves). Regrettably, despite the lethality of these risk factors, too frequently such behavior is not taken seriously, or minimized, even covered up by fellow officers. "It was only an accident," an officer said, after his partner took his service revolver, placed the gun to his head and shot himself. The officer said, "I saw the trigger pulled"; yet, he could not believe that it was a suicide.

Verbal Statements

As with behavior, the attitude toward individuals making verbal threats is too frequently negative. Statements are seen as "just for attention." This attitude results in ignoring the behavior of a person who is genuinely perturbed and potentially suicidal. This is true in the police; it is a blue world. The important question is, "Why this way of getting attention when there are so many other constructive ways?"

Examples of verbal warnings are the following: "I'm going to kill myself " or "If they take my gun, I'll kill myself," both being very direct. Other more indirect examples are the following: "I am going to see my (deceased) mother" or "I give up." Some other ways of expressing other-directed violence, are made in statements like, "People like the sergeant deserve to be dead."

Cognitive Clues

The single most frequent state of mind of the suicidal person is constriction (Hughes & Neimeyer, 1990). There is a tunnel vision, a narrowing of the mind's eye. There is a narrowing of the range of perception or opinions or options that occur to the mind. Frequently, the person uses words like "only," "always," "never," and "forever." The following are examples: "No one will ever love me. Only mom loved me"; "Sam was the only one who loved me"; "My ex-husband will always be that way"; and "Either I'll kill Sam or myself."

Emotional Clues

The person who is suicidal is often highly perturbed; he or she is disturbed, anxious, perhaps agitated. Depression, as already noted, is frequently evident. Suicidal people may feel boxed in, rejected, harassed, and unsuccessful. Some frequent feelings reported by patients are the following: anger, anxiety, emptiness, loneliness, loss, and sadness. A common emotional state in most suicidal people is hopelessness-helplessness. Statements like the following may signal hopelessness: "Nothing will change. Even the Chief rejected me. It will always be this way." Whereas helplessness may be verbalized as "There is nothing I can do. There is nothing my fellow officers can do to make a difference."

Sudden Behavioral Changes

Changes in behavior are also suspect. Both the outgoing individual who suddenly becomes depressed and isolated, and the normally reserved individual who starts being outgoing and drinking more, may be at risk. Such changes are of particular concern when a precipitating painful event is apparent. Changed performance at work may be an important clue. Reckless behavior, such as inappropriate displays of the gun or drinking at work or driving at high speeds in the patrol car may be clues. Making final arrangements such as giving away unusual personal belongings such as a service medal, a favorite firearm, or other possessions may be ominous (but is by no means a common clue, but may be in a specific case, of course). A preoccupation with death, such as reading and talking about death after the death of a loved one, may be a clue. Some people may suffer complicated grief; they do not overcome the loss of a loved one. They may be preoccupied with the death; they often identify with the dying person, and after the death, long for, even magically, a reunion. The death becomes the stimulus for believing that suicide is a solution, an escape from pain and grief. This loss is probably one of the most frequent and common stimuli to suicide around the world, including in officers. Nonetheless, constructive discussion or grief counseling after a death may not only be helpful for the individual but also essential. Education, a prevention, can help in the healing. There are so many possible behavioral cues and changes, not only about suicide, but also many red flags. One must evaluate the individual case, of course too; the unique. (Science can only tell us what evidence to look for, not what is in *this* major crime scene, whether suicide or homicide.)

Life-Threatening Behavior

The following are examples of life-threatening behavior often found in suicide. A 9-year veteran police officer, who had killed himself, had previously been seen leaning out of an open window at the police station, and, at another time, playing with his service gun. Following the rejection by his girlfriend, a 24-year-old male border-security service officer died in a single car accident on an isolated road after having had several similar accidents. A 70-year-old female, retired officer, with detailed knowledge of the Drug Unit of her police service, died from drug mismanagement, despite the nurse in her residence controlling her medication. Self-destruction is not rare. Often alcoholism, non-compliance with treatment, and inappropriate use of firearms can be seen in this light, as previously discussed. A verbal statement might be something like, "Who cares if I drink too much; the Sergeant; he drinks."

Suicide Notes

Like previous attempts and verbal statements, suicide notes are important clues; however, they are often read but not listened to by the reader. About 18% to 37% of adults leave notes (samples have varied greatly). There is no verifiable estimate available for police.

Here is a sample:

1. Adolf Hitler killed himself on April 30, 1945. Hitler is probably the perpetrator of the most homicides, followed by his suicide, in history worldwide. He wrote a last will on the 29th of April; there is no question in our mind that it is a genuine suicide note.

As I did not consider that I could take responsibility, during the years of struggle, of contracting a marriage, I have now decided, before the closing of my earthly career, to take as my wife that girl who, after many years of faithful friendship, entered, of her own free will the practically besieged town in order to share her destiny with me. At her own desire she goes as my wife with me into death. It will compensate us for what we both lost through my work in the service of my people.
What I possess belongs—in so far as it has any value—to the Party. Should this no longer exist, to the State; should the State also be destroyed, no further decision of mine is necessary.
My paintings, in the collections which I have bought in the course of years, have never been collected for private purposes, but only for the extension of a gallery in my home town of Linz on Donau.
It is my sincere wish that this bequest may be duly executed.
I nominate as my Executor my most faithful Party comrade,
Martin Bormann
He is given full legal authority to make all decisions.
He is permitted to take out everything that has a sentimental value or is necessary for the maintenance of a modest simple life, for my brothers and sisters, also above all for the mother of my wife and my faithful co-workers who are well known to him, principally my old Secretaries Frau Winter etc. Who have for many years aided me by their work.
I myself and my wife—in order to escape the disgrace of deposition or capitulation—choose death. It is our wish to be burnt immediately on the spot where I have carried out the greatest part of my daily work in the course of a twelve years' service to my people.

Given in Berlin, 29th April 1945, 4:00 A.M.
[Signed] A. Hitler

2. Kurt Cobain was a very famous, exceptionally talented rock star; his band, Nirvana, invented the grunge sound. Yet he painfully struggled; he had an emotional disturbance (psychopathology). On the 5th of April 1995, he shot himself. He is probably the most famous person who died by suicide in recent years. Here is his note:

To Boddah

Speaking from the tongue of an experienced simpleton who obviously would rather be an emasculated, infantile complain-ee. This note should be pretty easy to understand.

All the warnings from the punk rock 101 courses over the years, since my first introduction to the, shall we say, ethics involved with independence and the embracement of your community has proven to be very true. I haven't felt the excitement of listening to as well as creating music along with reading and writing for too many years now. I feel guilty beyond words about these things.

For example when we're back stage and the lights go out and the manic roar of the crowds begins, it doesn't affect me the way in which it did for Freddie

Mercury, who seemed to love, relish in the the love and adoration from the crowd which is something I totally admire and envy. The fact is, I can't fool you, any one of you. It simply isn't fair to you or me. The worst crime I can think of would be to rip people off by faking it and pretending as if I'm having 100% fun. Sometimes I feel as if I should have a punch-in time clock before I walk out on stage. I've tried everything within my power to appreciate it (and I do, God, believe me I do, but it's not enough). I appreciate the fact that I and we have affected and entertained a lot of people. It must be one of those narcissists who only appreciate things when they're gone. I'm too sensitive. I need to be slightly numb in order to regain the enthusiasms I once had as a child.

On our last 3 tours, I've had a much better appreciation for all the people I've known personally, and as fans of our music, but I still can't get over the frustration, the guilt and empathy I have for everyone. There's good in all of us and I think I simply love people too much, so much that it makes me feel too fucking sad. The sad little, sensitive, unappreciative, Pisces, Jesus man. Why don't you just enjoy it? I don't know!

I have a goddess of a wife who sweats ambition and empathy and a daughter who reminds me too much of what I used to be, full of love and joy, kissing every person she meets because everyone is good and will do her no harm. And that terrifies me to the point to where I can barely function. I can't stand the thought of Frances becoming the miserable, self-destructive, death rocker that I've become.

I have it good, very good, and I'm grateful, but since the age of seven, I've become hateful towards all humans in general. Only because it seems so easy for people to get along that have empathy. Only because I love and feel sorry for people too much I guess.

Thank you all from the pit of my burning, nauseous stomach for your letters and concern during the past years. I'm too much of an erratic, moody baby! I don't have the passion anymore, and so remember, it's better to burn out than to fade away.

Peace, love, empathy.
Kurt Cobain

Frances and Courtney, I'll be at your altar.
Please keep going Courtney,

for Frances
for her life which will be so much happier without me.

I LOVE YOU, I LOVE YOU!

3. Joe Smith, a homicide-suicide. He killed his children and wife, followed by his suicide. Here is his note:

Joe Smith, hold my father-in-law responsible for pressuring me to take the life of my wife and children. He is a killer. He plans and then causes trouble

> for us. I am taking the life of my wife and children because he is not worth that I should give my children to him.
>
> I said to you that the money is of no use to me. Now, be happy with your money.
>
> You bastard, you are a 3rd class person. You think that only the rich people speak the truth; sometimes you should see what you are doing.
>
> I, Joe Smith, in my full senses, do will the death of my wife, children, and me.

4. Moe Pergament was a suicide by cop (On this topic, the best book is Lindsay and Lester's, *Suicide By Cop* [2004]; see Chapter 2 in this volume). Officer Anthony Sica shot Moe. Here is Moe's suicide note to Officer Sica:

> Officer,
>
> It was a plan. I'm sorry to get you involved. I just needed to die. Please send my letters and break the news slowly to my family and let them know I had to do this. And that I love them very much. I'm sorry for getting you involved. Please remember that this was all my doing. You had no way of knowing.
>
> Moe Pargament

5. A 37-year-old police officer, wanting to kill his sergeant, but killed himself, wrote:

> Sergeant:
>
> Goodbye you old prick and when I mean prick you are a prick. Hope you fall with the rest of us, you yellow bastard.
>
> May precinct 25 get along without you.

Based on the discussion thus far, especially Clinical Observations and Behavioral Clues, a Suicide Lethality Checklist is presented in Table 1. It is a checklist of overt behavior; yet, as we will read next, such checklists have great limitations in predicting risk in people. However, before we proceed, we need to discuss evaluation of risk in general.

EVALUATION OF SUICIDE RISK

No one really knows how to assess suicide risk perfectly. One of the most frequent questions asked about suicide risk is, "How do you predict suicide risk?" or more specifically, the question in front of us is, "How do you assess or predict a police officer's suicide risk?" Indeed, suicide risk assessment may well be the most complex clinical task that psychiatrists, psychologists, GPs, and other mental health professionals face. The same is true for health professionals working with police officers. What is essential to learn is that assessment and prediction are interwoven with understanding. Could we have predicted the officer's suicide? Lt. Michael Pigott's? Kelly Johnson's?

In the 1960s and 1970s, there was a focus on the prediction of suicide, and suicidologists believed that it would eventually be possible to predict which individuals out of a population would ultimately complete suicide (Beck, Resnik, & Lettieri, 1974). However, it was soon realized that the statistical rarity of suicide and the imperfection of the prediction instruments led to an enormously large number of false positives; so many, in fact, that the prediction instruments were of little use to clinicians or to those planning suicide prevention services (Lester, 1974).

In the 1980s and 1990s, the focus shifted to assessment (Maris, Berman, Maltsberger, & Yufit, 1992). That is, rather than predicting the future occurrence of suicide in people, the intent was to assess potentially suicidal people in a more general sense, taking into account all of their life experiences; psychological characteristics; and specific culture, such as our blue one; which are relevant to future suicidal behavior (Maltsberger, 1986; Shneidman, 1985). Indeed, it is our belief that prediction and assessment are mutual processes and any separation is an artificial one. They are not separate categories.

Assessment requires clear definition. What is *it* that we are assessing? One value of the *Diagnostic and Statistical Manual of Mental Disorders, 4th Edition,* DSM, despite its many limitations, is that it teaches you to think in concise, standardized definitions of terms. This, as we learned from Shneidman (1985) is, however, complex.

In assessing suicide risk in people, we need to be aware of behaviors that are potentially predictive of suicide. However, there is no such definitive behavior. Suicide is a multidimensional event (Leenaars, 1988; Shneidman, 1980, 1985). Two concepts, which were introduced earlier and are essential in prediction, are *lethality* and *perturbation* (Shneidman, 1973, 1980, 1985, 1993).

There have been numerous attempts to construct tests for suicide prediction and related phenomena, most meeting with failure. In response to awareness of the inherent difficulties in predicting suicide, the National Institute of Mental Health (NIMH) of the United States organized a think tank for the assessment of suicidal behavior (Lewinsohn, Garrison, Langhinrichsen, & Marsteller, 1989). They reviewed all available assessment instruments used to study suicidal behavior. Their conclusion: *Few, if any, are useful.* Like each clue, each test, *by itself*, has little utility (Garrison, Lewinsohn, Marsteller, Langhinrichsen & Lann, 1991). Like in any forensic study, each clue, each test, each criterion, and so on has thus to be placed into the context of a larger array of facts. That is the basis of sound policing and science. Maris et al. (1992) reached the same conclusion, namely that one could not reduce the richness and diversity of suicide and destructive behavior to *the* test. Would one test have predicted an officer's suicide? Homicide-suicide?

Table 1. Suicide Lethality Checklist

Name ______________ Rater ______________ Date ______________

VERBAL STATEMENTS	LOW	MODERATE	HIGH
Plan	___ unplanned	___ general reference	___ specific reference
When	___ unclear	___ within few days, hours, etc.	___ immediate
Availability of means	___ unavailable	___ available-not preset	___ have in hand/used
Alcohol/drugs ingested	___ no		___ yes
Made final arrangements	___ vague	___ made some plans	___ given away possessions, will, etc.
PAIN	___ bearable		___ unbearable
PREVIOUS ATTEMPTS	___ none	___ one	___ multiple attempts
COGNITIVE – CONSTRICTION	___ none	___ some	___ marked
EMOTIONAL	___ appropriate emotional reactions to situations	___ appropriate and inappropriate	___ hopeless, helpless, ambivalence
SUICIDE NOTE	___ no		___ yes

DISORGANIZATION	___ none	___ confused	___ marked chaos
HEALTH (Describe)	___ no medical problems	___ moderate problems	___ chronic disability, learning disability, illness, weight loss, anorexia, sleep disorder
PRECIPITATING EVENT (especially if rejection/loss) (Describe)	___	___	___
SUDDEN BEHAVIOR (Describe)	___ none		___ marked
LIFE-THREATENING BEHAVIOR (e.g., alcohol/drug use) (Describe)	___	___	___
SOCIOEMOTIONAL PROBLEMS	___ infrequent	___ recent	___ chronic
WITHDRAWAL/ISOLATION	___ will accept help	___ hesitant to involve others	___ alone refuses help
SIGNIFICANT OTHERS	___ several available	___ few or only one	___ none

*Make notes on back (e.g., interpersonal relations, inability to adjust, indirection expressions, egression, ego).

Based on the discussion to this point, Table 1 presents a suicide lethality checklist, which is by no means a perfect one. Indeed, one can show very few behavioral clues, and even score at a low level of lethality on such a checklist and still be highly suicidal or homicidal-suicidal (see below, Dissembling: Clues to Suicide Reconsidered). Often officers, such as Chief Thomas Moffatt, showed no clues. No one predicted his suicide, a very common situation in suicide among police. Nonetheless, these clues may assist in many cases, since a large percentage of officers will show clues, but less than the 80% in the general population will. We, however, do not know what percentage. Of course, there is the old problem in policing and science, evidence or clues, say a suicide note, does not necessarily mean a suicide. There are false positives and true negatives (the real problem) (Leenaars, 1999b).

More comprehensive procedures such as the Thematic Guide for Suicide Prediction (TGSP) (Leenaars, 2004), to be presented later, may prove to be more useful in the future than specific measures, but there are not simple tools. These procedures are designed to assess a person's own narratives (stories), what the person says or writes in a suicide note or Internet writing (e-mails). Survivors too can help, a retrospective investigation (a psychological autopsy). These procedures are designed to measure the pain, lethality, and perturbation, and the psychology of suicide. It should be obvious, from a forensic view, that tests should not be used as a single basis or test for risk assessment, and a clinician, police officer, crisis worker, and so on, may have little utility for them in an individual case.

It is likely that no one behavior, including a test score or an interview, will provide all of the information needed to assess and predict suicide. An officer's suicide risk could not and cannot be assessed at one time by one test, one interview, or such. Each bit of information (like a test score, an observation) will have to be placed in the context of that person's life. It is likely that a number of tests, forensic clues, interviews and scales will be needed to predict such a complex human behavior as suicide, even retrospectively. No one test or behavior or observation may be the answer. This is not only because of the complexity, but also because of the low base (frequency) rate. There is no one "bump on the head" that will tell us whether an officer is suicidal or not, much less how suicidal that person is. Furthermore, all predictions ultimately depend on the skill of the clinician, police officer, and so on. In that sense, suicide prediction is a task like many others that an officer and clinician face: a problem of understanding a number of evaluations of the same person.

What would an officer's risk look like on the Suicide Lethality Checklist? On Beck's Suicide Intent Scale (BSIS) (Beck, Kovacs, & Weissman, 1975)? On Smith Lethality of Suicide Attempt Rating Scale (LSARS) (Smith, Conroy, & Ehler, 1984)? On Shneidman's list of predictive clues among the gifted Terman subjects who died by suicide (Shneidman, 1971)? On The Thematic Guide of Suicide Prediction (Leenaars, 2004)? What scale would help us? That is prediction. What scale, after the fact? This is postdiction.

SEX DIFFERENCES

The basic sex difference in suicide is that males kill themselves more than females do (although this is not so in China [Pritchard, 1996]). This is true in police. In contrast, females *attempt* suicide more often than males. This sex difference has been found in almost all nations (Lester, 1988a, 1992a). The male-female ratio of suicide has remained fairly stable over time. The generally accepted male-female ratio of completed suicides is 3 or 4 males to 1 female, but there is great variation around the world, and probably within police cultures.

Explanations in the literature (Leenaars, 1988) have varied. Females use different and less lethal methods (drugs vs. shooting). (Is this so for female officers? Probably, no.) Individuals with severe emotional disturbances (psychiatric disorders) have higher rates of suicide, and men are more likely to be diagnosed with such disorders. There are also alternative social expectations for men and women in trauma such that males act more catastrophically. Yet Shneidman (1985) has argued that genotypic similarities may be more prevalent than differences. Indeed, the author's research (Leenaars, 1988) on suicide notes of males and females confirms this. Pain is pain. Frustrated needs are frustrated needs. Constriction is constriction. Maybe there are phenotypic differences (e.g., method, diagnostic label) in suicide but not genotypic ones across sex. Could the high rates of completed suicide in males be more influenced by gender roles than psychological factors? Is this so in officers?

Tomlinson-Keasey, Warren, and Elliot (1986), in their study of gifted female suicides, came to the same conclusion as our study of notes. They found that the markers (e.g., emotional disturbance, a history of problems) of suicide were the same in both sexes. Others (e.g., Canetto, 1994; Canetto & Lester, 1995) have cited such factors as socioeconomic disadvantage, unemployment, domestic violence, and a history of suicidal behavior among friends and family as relevant to the suicides of women. Such factors have also been observed in the suicides of men (Lester, 1988a, 1992; Tomlinson-Keasey et al., 1986). The area is, however, plagued by stereotypes (Canetto, 1994). For example, the division of women's suicides as irrational and men's as rational is not supported in the data (Leenaars, 1988, 2004). Reflections on this topic are most relevant (Lester, 1988a). For example, if the officer who died by suicide was a female and women have significantly lower rates of suicide than men (and as you will learn extremely lower rates of homicide-suicide), maybe one should ask, Is the rate of suicide in female officers higher than the general population? Why did the female officer kill herself? Are the usual protective factors for females absent in female officers? Is the police culture a factor? Despite the research to date, are there unique factors in female suicide? Are there unique factors in female police officers' suicide? Are the critical factors the same as male officers? What factors are common and unique factors in female and male officers, who die by suicide? What about female officers' homicide-suicide, are they the same or different from male officers?

THEORY AND SUICIDE: A FOREWORD

As a crucial final point of introduction, there are, of course, views that theory should not play a role in understanding suicide. Suicidology should only be tabular and statistical. However, we believe that theory, explicit and implicit, plays a key role in understanding any behavior. Theory is the foundation in science (Kuhn, 1962). Newton, Einstein, Ferri, and all great scientists are great because they were theorists. It is only through theory, Edwin Shneidman (1985) once noted, that we will sort out the booming buzzing mess of experience (William James, 1890). In fact, it can be argued that "sciences have achieved their deepest and most far reaching insights by descending below the level of familiar empirical phenomena" (Hempel, 1966, p. 77). Theory may well be in the eye of the beholder (Kuhn, 1962), but it is pivotal in scientific understanding whether one is a researcher, police officer, or clinician. There is nothing as useful as good theory. People must make formulations about things to understand them (Husserl, 1907/1973). This does not mean that John Stuart Mill's set of basic rules for science (and, for that matter, for forensic investigation) have to be abandoned. In his *System of Logic,* Mill (1892/1984), reported a set of canons for inductively establishing causality. These are the Methods of Difference, of Agreement and Difference, of Residues, and of Concomitant Variation. In our study of police suicide, for example, Mill's Method of Difference does not need to be abandoned; as we will see, in fact, it will be essential. John Stuart Mill has answered many forensic questions. Thus, it would be wise to borrow the ideas of our leading theorists to answer empirically the question, "Why did officer kill herself? Why did he kill his spouse, followed by his suicide?"

A THEORY OF SUICIDE

Theory must begin with definition. Thus, again, let us offer the formal definition of suicide by Shneidman (1985):

> Currently in the Western world, suicide is a conscious act of self-induced annihilation, best understood as a multidimensional malaise in a needful individual who defines an issue for which suicide is perceived as the best solution. (p. 203)

Suicide is not simply a psychopathological entity in the DSM-IV (American Psychiatric Association, 1994). (It is actually only cited twice as a behavior; once under Depression and once under Borderline Personality Disorders.) We do not agree with those who point to an external stress as the sole cause of suicide. We also do not agree that it is only pain. We tend to place the emphasis on the multideterminant nature of suicide. Suicide is *intrapsychic*. It is stress and pain, but not simply the stress or even the pain, but the person's inability to cope with the event or pain. The issue of any schema about human personality is one that makes an individual an individual (Murray, 1938). It should be the study of the whole organism, not only the stress or pain. People do not simply commit suicide because of pain, but because it's unbearable; they are mentally constricted; they have a mental/emotional disorder; they cannot cope, and so on.

However, from a psychological view, suicide is not only intrapsychic, it is also *interpersonal* (or stated differently, it is both an inner and outer phenomenology). The suicidal individual is not only depressed, mentally constricted and so on, but also cut off from loved ones, ideals and even the community. The suicidal person is estranged. People live in a world (a society). Individuals are interwoven; the suicidal person, painfully so. We disagree with those who point to only some intrapsychic aspects such as anger turned inward or primitive narcissism to explain suicide. Suicide occurs in a person *and* between people (or some other ideal; e.g., being loved by someone, possession of the service revolver). This is not a Descartesian dichotomy; it is rather a dynamic interactional system. Yet the intrapsychic world is figural. Suicide occurs as a solution in a mind. The mentalistic processes are the foreground (such as the pain, depression). This is an important difference. It is in the inner world that a person makes the decision to jump, shoot, and so on. It is here that he decides, "This is the best solution." To put it simply: No drama, no stage. It is the intersection between the two phenomenologies that is essential to understand in suicide. It is, for example, not simply loss of the gun on the stage, but how the person's drama unfolds this very personal, individual stage. Metaphorically speaking, suicide is an intrapsychic drama on an interpersonal stage.

Two concepts, already discussed, that have been found to be essential and helpful in understanding the malaise are lethality and perturbation (Shneidman, 1973, 1980, 1985, 1993). Lethality refers to the probability of a person killing himself, and on quantification scales ranges from low to moderate to high. It is a psychological state of mind. Perturbation refers to subjective distress (disturbed, agitated, sane-insane), and can also be rated from low to moderate to high. Both concepts are needed to frame the following theory. It is important to note that one can be perturbed and not suicidal. Lethality kills, not perturbation.

To begin, suicide can be clinically understood from at least the following templates or patterns (Leenaars, 1988, 1989, 1995, 2004).

INTRAPSYCHIC DRAMA

1. Unbearable Psychological Pain

The common stimulus in suicide is *unbearable* psychological pain (Shneidman, 1985, 1993). The enemy of life is pain. The suicidal person is in a heightened state of perturbation, an intense mental anguish. This is what the author, William Styron (1990), called "The howling tempest of the brain." It is the pain of feeling pain. Although, as Menninger (1938) noted, other motives (elements, wishes) are evident, the person primarily wants to flee from pain experienced in a trauma, a catastrophe. The fear is that the trauma, the crisis is bottomless—an eternal suffering. The person may feel any number of emotions, such as boxed in, rejected, deprived, forlorn, distressed, and especially hopeless and helpless. It is the emotion of impotence, the feeling of being hopeless-helpless that is so painful for many suicidal people. The situation is unbearable and the person desperately wants a way out of it. The suicide, as Murray (1967) noted, is functional because it abolishes painful tension for the individual. It provides escape from intolerable suffering. Suicide is escape.

2. Cognitive Constriction

The common cognitive state in suicide is mental constriction (Shneidman, 1985). Constriction, that is, rigidity in thinking, narrowing of focus, tunnel vision, concreteness, and such, is the major component of the cognitive state in suicide. The person is figuratively "intoxicated" or "drugged" by the constriction; the intoxication can be seen in emotions, logic, and perception. The suicidal person exhibits at the moment before her death only permutations and combinations of a trauma (e.g., business failure, police scandal, poor health, and rejection by lover). The suicidal mind is in a special state of relatively fixed purpose and of relative constriction. In the face of the painful trauma, a possible solution became *the* solution. This constriction is one of the most dangerous aspects of the suicidal mind. (We highlight this more below.)

3. Indirect Expressions

Ambivalence, complications, redirected aggression, unconscious implications, and related indirect expressions (or phenomena) are often evident in suicide. The suicidal person is ambivalent. There are complications, concomitant contradictory feelings, attitudes, and thrusts, often toward a person and even toward life (See dissembling below). Not only is it love and hate but it may also be a conflict between survival and unbearable pain. The person experiences humility, submission, devotion, subordination, flagellation, and sometimes even masochism. Yet there is much more. What the person is conscious of is only a fragment of the suicidal mind (Freud, 1917a/1974). There are more reasons to the act than the suicidal person is consciously aware of when making the final decision (Freud, 1917a/1974; Freud, 1917b/1974; Leenaars, 1988, 1993b). The driving force may well be unconscious processes.

4. Inability to Adjust/Psychopathology

People with all types of pains, problems, and the like are at risk for suicide. Psychological autopsy studies suggest that 40% to 90% of people who kill themselves have some symptoms of psychopathology or problems in adjustment (Hawton & van Heeringen, 2000). As high as 60% appear to be related to mood disorders. Although the majority of suicides may, thus, fit best into mood nosological classifications, (e.g., depressive disorders, bipolar disorders, adjustment disorder with mixed anxiety and depressed mood), other emotional/mental disorders have been identified. For example, anxiety disorders (Post Traumatic Stress Disorder [PTSD] is especially prevalent in police), schizophrenic disorders (especially paranoid type), panic disorders, borderline personality disorders, antisocial personality disorders have been related to suicides (Leenaars, 1988; Sullivan, 1962, 1964). Anxiety may well be an equally important pain, next to depression (Fawcett, 1997). Schizophrenics have a very high rate (about 5%, not the often-cited 10%) (Palmer, Pankratz, & Bostwick, 2005). Yet there are other disorders not specified that may result in risk. From the autopsy data, it is learned that many may have no disorder identifiable in DSM-IV (or some other classification scheme, such as ICD). The person may be simply paralyzed by pain that life, a future, or such are colorless and unattractive.

Depression, in its varieties, is however, the most frequent disorder; however, it must be understood by any reader that not all suicidal people are depressed, and that not all depressed people are suicidal. It is often cited that 15% of people who develop depression ultimately kill themselves. Bostwick (2000) has, however, clearly demonstrated in a meta-analysis of the research that this is a myth. It may well, in fact, be as low as 2%. Most important, it is important to remember that suicidal people experience unbearable pain, not always depression, and even if they do experience depression, the critical stimulus is the unbearable nature of the depression (as in some other mood). Suicidal people see themselves as in unendurable pain and unable to adjust. His state of mind is, however, incompatible with accurate discernment of what is going on. Having the belief that they are too weak to overcome difficulties, these people reject everything except death—they do not survive life's difficulties.

5. Ego

The ego, with its enormous complexity (Murray, 1938), is an essential factor in the suicidal scenario. The OED defines ego as "the part of the mind that reacts to reality and has a sense of individuality." Ego strength is a protective factor against suicide. The biological perspective has equally argued this conclusion; van Praag (1997) has, for example, clearly documented a biological aspect to suicidal people, such as increased susceptibility to stressors, labile anxiety, and aggression regulation. Suicidal people frequently exhibit a relative weakness in their capacity to develop constructive tendencies and to overcome their personal difficulties (Zilboorg, 1936). The person's ego has likely been weakened by a steady toll of traumatic life events (e.g., loss, rejection, abuse, demotion, transfer to a perceived lesser department [a "promotion"]). This implies that a history of traumatic disruptions—*pain*—placed the person at risk for suicide; it likely mentally or emotionally handicapped the person's ability to develop mechanisms (or ego functions) to cope. There is, to put it in one simple word, vulnerability. There is a lack of resilience. A weakened ego correlates positively with suicide risk.

INTERPERSONAL STAGE

6. Interpersonal Relations

The suicidal person has problems in establishing or maintaining relationships. There frequently is a disturbed, unbearable interpersonal situation. A calamity prevailed. A positive development in those same disturbed relationships may have been seen as the only possible way to go on living, but such development was seen as not forthcoming. The person's psychological needs are frustrated. Suicide appears to be related to an unsatisfied or frustrated attachment need, although other needs, often more intrapsychic, may be equally evident, for example, achievement, autonomy, dominance, honor. Suicide is committed because of thwarted or unfulfilled needs, needs that are often frustrated interpersonally.

The possible needs that are frustrated or blocked are expansive. Here is a partial list of needs, adopted from Henry A. Murray's *Explorations in Personality* (1938):

Abasement. To submit passively to external force; accept injury, criticism, punishment; to surrender; become resigned to fate; blame or belittle self.

Achievement. To accomplish something difficult; master, manipulate, organize physical objects, human beings or ideas; to overcome; to excel oneself.

Affiliation. To enjoyably cooperate or reciprocate with an allied other; to please and win affection; to adhere or remain loyal to a friend or group.

Aggression. To overcome opposition forcefully; to fight; to attack or injure another; to oppose forcefully or punish other.

Autonomy. To get free, shake off restraint; break out of social confinement; avoid or quit activities of domineering authorities; be independent and free.

Counteraction. To make up for failure by restriving; overcome weakness or repress fear; to maintain self-respect and pride on a high level; overcome.

Defendance. To defend or vindicate the self against assault, criticism, blame; conceal or justify a misdeed, failure or humiliation.

Deference. To admire and support a superior; praise, honor or eulogize; yield eagerly to influence of another; emulate an exemplar.

Dominance. To control other humans; influence or direct others by command, suggestion or persuasion; or to dissuade, restrain or prohibit others.

Exhibition. To make an impression; be seen and heard; to excite, amaze, fascinate, entertain, shock, intrigue, amuse, or entice others.

Harm avoidance. To avoid pain, physical injury, illness, and death; escape from a dangerous situation; to take precautionary measures.

Infavoidance. To avoid humiliation; avoid or quit conditions that lead to scorn, derision, indifference or embarrassment.

Inviolacy. To protect the self; remain separate; maintain distance; to resist others' intrusion on one's own psychological space; isolated.

Nurturance. To gratify the needs of another person, especially one who is weaker; to feed, help, support, console, protect, comfort; to nurture.

Order. To put things or ideas in order; to achieve arrangement, balance, organization, tidiness and precision among things and ideas.

Play. To act for fun. To enjoy relaxation of stress; to laugh and make jokes; to seek pleasurable activities for their own sake.

Rejection. To exclude, abandon, expel, separate oneself or remain indifferent to a negatively seen person; to snub or jilt another.

Sentience. To seek and enjoy sensuous experience; to give an important place to creature comforts and satisfaction of the senses—taste, touch.

Succorance. To have one's needs gratified by the sympathetic aid of another; be supported, sustained, guided, consoled, taken care of; protected.

Understanding. To ask questions; be interested in theory; speculate, analyze, generalize; to want to know the answers.

What were the needs of officers who died by suicide?

7. Rejection-Aggression

The rejection-aggression hypothesis was first documented by Wilhelm Stekel in the famous 1910 meeting of the Psychoanalytic Society in Freud's home in Vienna (Friedman, 1910/1967b). Adler, Jung, Freud, Sullivan, and Zilboorg have all expounded variations of this hypothesis. Loss is central to suicide; it is, in fact, often a rejection that is experienced as an abandonment. It is an unbearable narcissistic injury. This injury is part of a traumatic event that leads to pain and in some, self-directed aggression. In the first controlled study of suicide notes, Shneidman and Farberow (1957) reported, for example, that both hate directed toward others and self-blame are evident in notes. The suicidal person is deeply ambivalent and, within the context of this ambivalence, suicide may become the turning back upon oneself of murderous impulses (wishes, needs) that had previously been directed against a traumatic event, most frequently someone who had rejected that individual. Biological research in the field has demonstrated a neurobiological link between aggression and suicide. Despite a minimizing of this fact by some (e.g., Shneidman, 1985), aggression, whether other or self-directed, has for example, an association to serotonin dysfunction (Asberg et al., 1976). Freud's hypothesis appears to have a biological basis within the biopsychosocial view of suicide. Aggression is, in fact, a common emotional state in suicide. Suicide may be veiled aggression—it may be murder turned 180 degrees (Shneidman, 1985).

8. Identification-Egression

Freud (1917a/1974, 1920/1974, 1921/1974) hypothesized that intense identification with a lost or rejecting person or, as Zilboorg (1936) showed, with any lost ideal (e.g., health, promotion, employment, gun ownership) is crucial in understanding the suicidal person (police officer). Identification is defined as an attachment (bond), based upon an important emotional tie with another person (object) (Freud, 1920/1974) or any ideal. If this emotional need is not met, the suicidal person experiences a deep pain (discomfort). There is an intense desperation and the person wants to egress, that is, to escape. Something must be done to stop the anguish. The suicidal person wants to leave, to exit, to get out, to get away, to be gone, to be elsewhere . . . to not be . . . to be dead. Suicide becomes the only solution, and the person plunges into the abyss. *Suicide is escape*.

In concluding, the theory outlined is only one point of view. Yet the elements have utility in understanding suicide. Indeed, to begin to address the question, "Why do people kill themselves?" or more specifically, "Why did the officer commit suicide?" we need a psychology of suicide (and also, of homicide-suicide). We must answer the question, What are the important common psychological dimensions of suicide?—rather than, What kind of people commit suicide? The question is critical, for these common dimensions (or "samenesses") are what suicide is. Not necessarily the universal, but certainly the most frequent or common characteristics provide us with a meaningful conceptualization of suicide.

Research on Theory: An Empirically Based Understanding

Understanding the act of suicide and motives behind suicide behavior seems extremely important worldwide (WHO, 2002), and in order to do so empirically, many researchers from around the world have used different methods. Shneidman and Farberow (1957), Maris (1981), and others have suggested the following avenues: national mortality statistics, retrospective psychological investigations (often called psychological autopsies), the study of nonfatal suicide attempts and the analysis of documents (such as suicide notes). All of them have their limitations, and there are problems in obtaining them in many countries, including in subpopulations such as police officers. Yet each of these methods has been shown to extend our understanding of suicide and suicidal behavior (Hawton & van Heeringen, 2000; Leenaars et al., 1997). We will next examine the theory in the *prime facia* evidence in cases of suicide, and by implication, homicide-suicide, suicide notes (Leenaars, 1999b).

Early research (e.g., de Boismont, 1856; Wolff, 1931) on suicide notes largely used an anecdotal approach that incorporated descriptive information (Frederick, 1969). Subsequent methods, using Frederick's (1969) scheme for methods of analysis have used content analysis, classification analysis, and theoretical-conceptual analysis. Each of these approaches has had utility, although Frederick suggested that simple content analysis has limitations (see, for example, Ogilvie, Stone, & Shneidman, 1969; they noted that the word "love" occurs frequently in suicide notes). Classification schemes use data such as age, sex, marital status, educational level, employment status, and mental disorder (see, for example, Ho, Yip, Chiu, & Halliday, 1998). Ho and his colleagues (1998) developed the most widely used classification scheme; they studied suicides notes in Hong Kong. Ho's scheme is largely based on forensic data that are gathered at post-mortem investigation. They found that suicide notes written by young people were longer and richer in emotions than those written by older people. A similar classification scheme has been used in India (Girdhar, Leenaars, Dogra, Leenaars, & Kumar, 2004), Mexico (Chavez, Paramo-Castello, Leenaars, & Leenaars, 2006), and Turkey (Demirel, Akar, Sayin, Candansayar, & Leenaars, 2008). However, as Girdhar and her team noted, there are limitations. The data are not entirely consistent, and differences in collection occur between researchers in different countries. There are also limitations in the generalizability of the findings. For example, unlike Ho's finding, Demirel and the team from Turkey found the notes from the elderly longer. For a further example, Girdhar's team from India found that many notes involved a specific instruction, mostly for care of the family; physical/psychological illness was the most frequently mentioned difficulty; whereas Chavez and her group from Mexico found little written about life's difficulties and few specific instructions. Furthermore, a comparison of note writers with non–note writers, has failed to find consistent results (Girdhar et al., 2004; Ho et al., 1998). Differences of demographic features like age and sex are also inconsistent (Chavez et al., 2006; Foster, 2003; Ho et al., 1998). Yet the studies have also supported the value of the data and the notion that suicide is complex (Ho et al., 1998; Leenaars, 1988; Shneidman & Farberow, 1957), warranting, among other things, more in-depth study of suicide notes in different cultures.

Only a very few studies have utilized a theoretical-conceptual analysis (Frederick, 1969), despite the assertion in the first formal study of suicide notes (Shneidman & Farberow, 1957) and in ongoing discussion (Diamond, More, Hawkins, & Soucar, 1995) that such an approach offers much promise. To address this lack, over 30 years ago, the author applied a logical, empirical analysis to suicide notes. The method permits a theoretical analysis of suicide notes, augments the effectiveness of controls, and allows us to develop some theoretical insight into the vexing problem of suicide that may have cross-cultural application.

The method has been previously described in detail (Leenaars, 1988; 2004; Leenaars & Balance, 1984). It treats suicide notes as an archival source. This source is subjected to the scrutiny of control hypotheses, following an *ex post facto* research design (Kerlinger, 1964). The major problem with the current type of research is the lack of control over extraneous variables and the large number of potentially important antecedent variables; thus, the danger of misinterpreting relationships. Kerlinger (1964) suggested that these problems could be largely overcome by explicitly formulating not just a single hypothesis, but several "control" hypotheses as well. This would call for suicide protocol, such as notes to be recast in different theoretical contexts (hypotheses, theories, models) for which lines of evidence of each of these positions can then be pursued in the data. Carnap's (1931/1959) logical and empirical procedures can be utilized for such investigations. To date, the theories of 10 suicidologists, as noted earlier, have been investigated: Alfred Adler, Ludwig Binswanger, Sigmund Freud, Carl Gustav Jung, Karl A. Menninger, Geroge Kelly, Henry A. Murray, Edwin S. Shneidman, Harry Stack Sullivan, and Gregory Zilboorg. In order to test the formulations, Carnap's (1931/1959) positivistic procedure calls for the translating of theoretical formulations into observable (specific) protocol sentences (Ayer, 1959).

To summarize from the world's largest array of empirical studies on suicide notes (e.g., age, sex, method used, nation) of the theories of the 10 suicidologists, a number of theoretical propositions/implications (or protocol sentences) have been identified to be observable in various samples of notes, the very words of a suicidal person. In the model, Leenaars isolated 10 protocol sentences from each of the ten theorists ($n = 100$) and reduced them to 35 sentences; 23 protocol sentences were found to be highly predictive (described) for the content of suicide notes (i.e., one standard deviation above the mean of observations), and 17 protocol sentences significantly discriminated genuine suicide notes from simulated notes (i.e., control data) (with 5 sentences being both) (Leenaars & Balance, 1984; Leenaars, 1989). One unique finding of these studies is that there are considerable age differences in the suicide notes, but not sex (Leenaars, 2004; Leenaars, de Wilde, Wenckstern, & Kral, 2001). Using Cluster Analysis, the protocols were reduced to the eight clusters discussed previously, grouped in 5 intrapsychic and 3 interpersonal aspects: (1) unbearable pain, (2) cognitive constriction, (3) indirect expressions, (4) inability to adjust (psychopathology), (5) ego (vulnerability), (6) interpersonal relationships, (7) rejection-aggression, and (8) identification-egression (Leenaars, 1996, 2004; Leenaars et al., 2001). Further, from a series of studies, Leenaars (1988, 1996) proposed a metaframe to organize the clusters into *intrapsychic* and *interpersonal* elements. Suicide can be, in fact, seen as an intrapsychic drama on an interpersonal stage. Suicide can, thus, be theoretically understood from the proposed theory (templates, constructs, and frames), outlined earlier in detail. There is, without a doubt, evidence for the theory, having great utility not only for research, but also for policing.

Table 2 presents the actual protocol sentences within each cluster, presented as a Thematic Guide for Suicide Prediction, TGSP. To apply the TGSP to each of the suicide notes presented earlier, we present the actual scores. (The reader may wish to do so):

1. Adolf Hitler's note:
   1, 2, 3, 4, 6, 7, 9, 12, 13, 15g, 17, 19, 20, 21, 23, 25, 26, 27, 29, 30, 31, 32, 33, 34, 35.
2. Kurt Cobain's note:
   1, 2, 3, 4, 5, 6, 7, 8, 9, 10, 11, 12, 13, 14, 15f, 16, 17, 18, 19, 20, 21, 22, 23, 24, 25, 26, 27, 28, 33, 34, 35.
3. Joe Smith's homicide-suicide note:
   1, 2, 3, 4, 6, 7, 8, 9, 11, 12, 13, 14, 15g, 17, 20, 21, 22, 25, 26, 27, 29, 30, 31, 32, 33, 34, 35.
4. Moe Pergament's note:
   1, 2, 3, 4, 5, 6, 8, 9, 11, 12, 13, 15g, 16, 18, 20, 21, 24, 25, 26, 29, 31, 32, 34, 35.
5. The police officer's note to the Sergeant (also found on the cover of this book):
   1, 2, 3, 6, 7, 8, 9, 12, 27, 29, 30, 31, 32, 35.

Independent research on suicide notes (O'Connor, Sheeby, & O'Connor, 1999), investigation of suicidal Internet writing (Barak & Miran, 2005), and biographical studies of suicides (Lester, 1994) have supported the utility of the approach to note, or any narrative, analysis. Barak and Miran (2005) found that unbearable pain, cognitive constriction, and problematic interpersonal relationships were especially evident in writings on the Internet about suicide; Lester (1994) found evidence of all aspects of Leenaars' model in the biographies of people who died by suicide. In-depth studies of interjudge reliability (for example, O'Connor et al., 1999) and over three decades of study by the author and colleagues show that, indeed, the percentage of interjudge agreement has been satisfactory (> 85%; see Shaughnessy, Zechmeister, & Zechmeister, 2000). Reliability and validity have also been established in different countries.

International studies are not only rare in the study of suicide notes, but suicide in general. There are only a few studies, for example, on suicide notes from different countries. Given that Canada has a higher rate of suicide than the United States (Leenaars & Lester, 1994b), Leenaars (1992) examined 56 suicide notes from Canada and the United States, whose writers were matched for age and sex (this was the first cross-cultural study of suicide notes). None of the intrapsychic or interpersonal aspects differed. Subsequently, studies from Germany (Leenaars, Lester, Wenckstern & Heim, 1994), United Kingdom (O'Connor & Leenaars, 2004), Hungary (Leenaars, Fekete, Wenckstern, & Osvath, 1998), Russia (Leenaars, Lester, Lopatin, Schustov, & Wenckstern, 2002), Australia (Leenaars, Haines, Wenckstern, Williams, & Lester, 2003), India (Leenaars,

Table 2.
THEMATIC GUIDE FOR SUICIDE PREDICTION
Antoon A. Leenaars, Ph.D., C.Psych.

I PATIENT DATA

Date: ____________________

Name ______________________________________ Age _____ Sex ____

Date of Birth ___________ --- ________________ Marital Status ___ Divorced ___

Education Status ______________ (years) __________________ (degrees)

Current Employment ____

II SUICIDAL EXPERIENCE

1) Has the patient ever seriously contemplated suicide? (If yes, note particulars)

____

2) Has the patient ever attempted suicide? (If yes, note particulars)

____

3) Does the patient know anyone who attempted suicide? (If yes, indicate family, acquaintance, etc.)

____

4) Does the patient know anyone who committed suicide? (If yes, indicate family, acquaintance, etc.)

____

III REFERRAL DATA

1) Purpose ____________________ Postvention ___________________________

2) What is the referral question? _______ See file _________________________

____

3) What is the presenting problem(s)? ____ See file ______________________

____

____

Table 2. (Cont'd.)

IV INTERVIEW SITUATION

1) Observations ______________________________

2) Other procedures (e.g., tests, interviews) ______________________________

V INTERPRETATIONS

	Low	Medium	High
1) Perturbation rating:	Low	Medium	High
scale equivalent	1 2 3	4 5 6	7 8 9
2) Lethality rating:	Low	Medium	High
scale equivalent	1 2 3	4 5 6	7 8 9

3) Guide summary:
scores: I – 1, 2, 3, 4, 5, 6; II – 7, 8, 9; III – 10, 11, 12;
IV – 13, 14, 15; V – 16, 17, 18; VI – 19, 20, 21, 22, 23, 24
VII – 25, 26, 27, 28, 29, 30, 31, 32; VII – 33, 34, 35

Conclusions: ______________________________

VI REMARKS

____

Include on back any other relevant data.

Table 2. (Cont'd.)

INSTRUCTIONS

Your task will be to verify whether the statements provided below correspond or compare with the contents of the patient's protocols (e.g., interview, written reports). The statements provided below are a classification of the possible content. You are to determine whether the contents in the patient's protocols are a particular or specific instance of the classification or not. Your comparison should be observable; however, the classification may be more abstract than the specific instances. Thus, you will have to make judgments about whether particular contents of a protocol are included in a given classification or not. Your task is to conclude, yes or no.

INTRAPSYCHIC	Circle One
I – Unbearable Psychological Pain	
1) Suicide has adjustive value and is functional because it stops painful tension and provides relief from intolerable psychological pain. (P)*	Yes No
2) In suicide, the psychological and/or environmental traumas among many other factors may include: incurable disease, threat of senility, fear of becoming hopelessly dependent, feelings of inadequacy, humiliation. Although the solution of suicide is not caused by one thing, or motive, suicide is a flight from these specters. (P & D)	Yes No
3) In the suicidal drama, certain emotional states are present, including pitiful forlornness, emotional deprivation, distress and/or grief. (P & D)	Yes No
4) The suicidal person (S) appears to have arrived at the end of an interest to endure and sees suicide as a solution for some urgent problem(s), and/or injustices of life. (P)	Yes No
5) There is a conflict between life's demands for adaptation and and the S's inability or unwillingness to meet the challenge. (P)	Yes No
6) S is in a state of heightened disturbance (perturbation) and feels boxed in, harassed, especially hopeless and helpless. (P)	Yes No

*The letter P refers to a specific highly predictive variable, whereas the letter D refers to a specific differentiating variable of the suicidal mind.

Table 2. (Cont'd.)

II – Cognitive Constriction	
7) S reports a history of trauma (e.g., poor health, rejection by significant other, a competitive spouse). (P & D)	Yes No
8) Figuratively speaking, S appears to be "intoxicated" by overpowering emotions. Concomitantly, there is a constricted logic and perception. (D)	Yes No
9) There is poverty of thought, exhibited by focusing only on permutations and combinations of grief and grief-provoking topics. (D)	Yes No
III – Indirect Expressions	
10) S reports ambivalence; e.g., complications, concomitant contradictory feelings, attitudes and/or thrusts. (P & D)	Yes No
11) S's aggression has been turned inwards; for example, humility, submission and devotion, subordination, flagellation, masochism are evident. (P)	Yes No
12) Unconscious dynamics can be concluded. There are likely more reasons to the suicide than the person is consciously aware. (D)	Yes No
IV – Inability to Adjust	
13) S considers him/herself too weak to overcome personal difficulties and, therefore, rejects everything, wanting to escape painful life events. (P)	Yes No
14) Although S passionately argues that there is no justification for living on, S's state of mind is incompatible with an accurate assessment/perception of what is going on. (P)	Yes No
15) S exhibits a serious disorder in adjustment. (P)	Yes No
a) S's reports are consistent with a manic-depressive disorder such as the down-phase; e.g., all-embracing negative statements, severe mood disturbances causing marked impairment.	Yes No
b) S's reports are consistent with schizophrenia; e.g., delusional thought, paranoid ideation.	Yes No

Table 2. (Cont'd.)

c) S's reports are consistent with anxiety disorder (such as obsessive-compulsive, posttraumatic stress); e.g., feeling of losing control; recurrent and persistent thoughts, impulses or images.	Yes	No
d) S's reports are consistent with antisocial personality (or conduct) disorder; e.g., deceitfulness, conning others.	Yes	No
e) S's reports are consistent with borderline personality disorder; e.g., frantic efforts to avoid real or imagined abandonment, unstable relationships.	Yes	No
f) S's reports are consistent with depression; e.g., depressed mood, diminished interest, insomnia.	Yes	No
g) S's reports are consistent with a disorder not otherwise specified. S is so paralyzed by pain that life, future, etc. is colorless and unattractive.		
V – Ego		
16) There is a relative weakness in S's capacity for developing constructive tendencies (e.g., attachment, love). (D)	Yes	No
17) There are unresolved problems ("a complex" or weakened ego) in the individual; e.g., symptoms or ideas that are discordant, unassimilated, and/or antagonistic. (P)	Yes	No
18) S reports that the suicide is related to a harsh conscience; i.e., a fulfillment of punishment (or self-punishment). (D)	Yes	No
INTERPERSONAL		
VI – Interpersonal Relations		
19) S's problem(s) appears to be determined by the individual's history and the present interpersonal situation. (P)	Yes	No
20) S reports being weakened and/or defeated by unresolved problems in the interpersonal field (or some other ideal such as health, perfection). (P)	Yes	No

Table 2. (Cont'd.)

21)	S's suicide appears related to unsatisfied or frustrated needs; e.g., attachment, perfection, achievement, autonomy, control. (P)	Yes No
22)	S's frustration in the interpersonal field is exceedingly stressful and persisting to a traumatic degree. (P)	Yes No
23)	A positive development in the disturbed relationship was seen as the only possible way to go on living, but such development was seen as not forthcoming. (P)	Yes No
24)	S's relationships (attachments) were too unhealthy and/or too intimate (regressive, "primitive"), keeping him/her under constant strain of stimulation and frustration. (D)	Yes No
VII – Rejection – Aggression		
25)	S reports a traumatic event or hurt or injury (e.g., unmet love, a failing marriage, disgust with one's work). (P)	Yes No
26)	S, whose personality (ego) is not adequately developed (weakened), appears to have suffered a narcissistic injury. (P & D)	Yes No
27)	S is preoccupied with an event or injury, namely a person who has been lost or rejecting (i.e., abandonment). (D)	Yes No
28)	S feels quite ambivalent, i.e., both affectionate and hostile toward the same (lost or rejection) person. (D)	Yes No
29)	S reports feelings and/or ideas of aggression and vengefulness toward him/herself, although S appears to be actually angry at someone else. (D)	Yes No
30)	S turns upon the self, murderous impulses that had previously been directed against someone else. (D)	Yes No
31)	Although maybe not reported directly, S may have calculated the self-destructiveness to have a negative effect on someone else (e.g., a lost or rejecting person). (P)	Yes No
32)	S's self-destructiveness appears to be an act of aggression, attack, and/or revenge toward someone else who has hurt or injured him/her. (P)	Yes No

Table 2. (Cont'd.)

VIII – Identification – Egression		
33)	S reports in some direct or indirect fashion an identification (i.e., attachment) with a lost or rejecting person (or with any lost ideal [e.g., health, freedom, employment, all A's]). (D)	Yes No
34)	An unwillingness to accept the pain of losing an ideal (e.g., abandonment, sickness, old age), allows S to choose, even seek to escape from life and accept death. (D)	Yes No
35)	S wants to egress (i.e., to escape, to depart, to flee, to be gone), to relieve the unbearable psychological pain. (P)	Yes No

Girdhar, Dogra, Wenckstern, & Leenaars, 2009), Mexico (Chavez, Leenaars, Chavez-de Sanchez, & Leenaars, 2009), and Turkey (Sayin et al., 2009) supported this observation. A few differences, however, were observed in some people: some cultural/social groups showed more indirect expressions, such as unconscious processes, ambivalence, and dissembling, and some more interpersonal elements of aggression, murderous impulses, and revenge, to an *Othello* rage (Leenaars, 2007). (And this, by implication, will be true in some officers, for cultural or many other reasons, to be discussed). There are differences by age; younger officers will show more mental constriction, being absolutely singularly focused on a reprimand, being arrested; that is, one single problem. One often sees relationships figural to them. Yet the theory has been empirically applicable to all people. Thus, the model has significant cross-cultural or social application; be that as it may, questions remain. Does it apply to subcultures, such as suicide in police officers? Probably. (Police services do not release suicide notes to allow for nomothetic study. What does Lt. Michael Pigott's note say?)

The history of suicidology (psychiatry, psychology, sociology, and so on) gives us the ideas, concepts, formulations, and so on, and science gives us the observable "valid" ones. This is the best of all possible psychologies, an empirically supported one. The theory outlined is an attempt to do that. There are few such theories in suicidology. It provides an answer to the question posed; it presents some common elements to answer why the police officer killed himself.

These elements, common to suicide, highlight that suicide is not only due to external stress or pain or even unattachment. The common consistency in suicide is, in fact, lifelong adjustment patterns (Shneidman, 1985). Suicidal people have experienced a steady toll of life events—threat, stress, failure, loss and challenge, or in one word, pain—that has undermined their ability to cope. Suicide has a history. The officer's homicide-suicide has a history.

Hopefully, the synthesis here presented will provide a useful clinical and forensic perspective for many on the question, "Why did the officer commit homicide-suicide?" and, as we will see later on the question, "How do we prevent such events in the future with suicidal police officers?"

Of course, we do not know whether the theory applies to all suicides. Suicide bombers, homicides-suicides, suicide martyrs, altruistic suicides, for example, may differ (Leenaars & Wenckstern, 2004). Today we have Islamic extremists who, cognitively constricted to the point of being delusional, in the glory of Allah, kill "infidels" and themselves; a homicide-suicide. There are many different kinds of homicide-suicides. Not so long ago, we had the Korean and Vietnamese monks who burned themselves for democratic freedom and independence from American tyranny. There is a long history, the Christian martyrs being one example. Yet we do not know whether these suicides and homicides-suicides are the same or different. We recently published the first study in the world on the writings of suicide martyrs. We (Leenaars, Parks, Collins, Wenckstern, & Leenaars, 2009) examined 33 letters of "altruistic suicides" and compared them blindly with a matched sample of the more "common" suicides (J. S. Mill's methods of difference and of agreement or similarity). We answer some key questions: Are suicide martyrs the same or different than suicide? What intra-psychic elements are critical for predicting a would-be martyr to kill herself? To kill you? Are interpersonal protocols relevant? What elements? Is ambivalence salient? There are many unique insights offered by the personal documents (e.g., martyrs' last letters, Internet writings) of suicide bombers. This is the topic of, as we will learn in the next chapter, the variety of homicide-suicides. Is the suicide bomber and a homicide-suicide of a police officer related?

On the topic of the suicide terrorist, Maltsberger (2001) insightfully speculated,

> One day a messianic leader, inflamed with malignant narcissistic fury, will become so intoxicated with the desire for revenge and destruction of his enemies that he will no longer be deterred by any self-preservative instinct or compassion for the welfare of his own people. Herman Melville imagined such a leader in Captain Ahab, who so nursed his grievance against Moby Dick, the white whale that bit off his leg, that he destroyed himself and his entire crew in his quest for revenge. (p. 145)

Is the officer who died by suicide, a Captain Ahab? Did he have grandiose fury? Is she an Othello?

A NOTE ON THE COGNITIVE STYLE

The best known faulty syllogism may well be,

> All men are immortal
> Socrates is a man
> Therefore Socrates is immortal.

The above syllogism is valid, but it is also faulty because it begins with a first premise that is false. It is a false universal inductive generalization. It is basic to realize that a valid syllogism can have a false conclusion. This can happen if one or more of the premises are false (Kahane, 1973). And in the suicidal person, the first premise (sometimes called core beliefs) is not only false, but also lethal.

Edwin Shneidman (Leenaars, 1993a, 1999b) has been keenly interested in making explicit the latent logical (cognitive) components of everyday thought. Later, he realized how useful it is to examine the cognitive styles exhibited in *each* suicidal person. For example, in a terse but insightful paper, "On 'Therefore I must kill myself'" (Shneidman, 1999), he shows how vitally important it is for a clinician to understand the patient's idiosyncratic logical style—and then not agree with that patient's major premise when the premise is the keystone to the patient's lethal (suicidal) syllogistic conclusion. For example, "People who have committed a certain sin ought to be dead; I am a person who has committed that sin; *therefore*, I ought to be dead." For another example, "People who are rejected by someone ought to be dead. I am a person who has been rejected; *therefore*, I ought to be dead." For another example, "People who kill ought to be dead. I am a person who killed; *therefore*, I ought to be dead." The homicidal mind is often the same. "People who abandon me ought to be dead. I am a person who has been abandoned. Therefore, he ought to be dead." The collaboration of the two, a suicide and a homicide, is even more lethal. This means that people need to know the suicidal person's mind, and the homicidal-suicidal person's mind. Only one is too limiting. Therefore, you have to know what suicide is. Further, if you do, you will not agree with the cognition, the major premise, "People who are rejected by the Chief ought to be dead," or some other *lethal* premise (or belief).

Yet we, akin to Shneidman (1999), think that the logic is wrong. It all depends on the word "therefore." It is perhaps the most important word in life and, it seems, death. When we invoke the word "therefore," we have come to a decision or resolution. Therefore, it is the pivotal word in logic, specifically, syllogisms. Shneidman (1999) writes,

> We all know that there are bridge-words between thought and action. Words like "might," "ought," "should," "must"—which convey *various* amounts of psychological *push*. The point is that *not all "therefores" are psychologically identical*, or to put it another way: not all equal signs are equally equal. Thus the word "therefore" cannot be taken for granted as a word which means "always" or "under all circumstances" as in the syllogism about Socrates. In *that* example, Socrates is *always* mortal, but that example simply illustrates the confinements of traditional Aristotelian syllogisms. (p. 74)

Yet there is an even more important fact, the mind does much more than simply logic. The sinner is an example. The sinner makes the classical error; the major premise is false. All humans are not immortal. And all people who have committed a certain sin ought not to be dead. What were the cognitions, premises, beliefs, and so on of the officer who died by suicide?

Once you know what suicide is, we believe that it is easy to conclude the following: The suicidal person, at the moment of taking his life, is figuratively intoxicated with his overpowering emotions and constricted logic. Are these suicidal people rational? Was the officer rational?

Cognitive constriction is an essential element of the suicidal mind. It is imperative that the reader be reminded that the suicidal person defines the trauma. A trauma is a perception, not a thing in itself. This was true for Othello. An educational example of Shneidman's is the man who always wanted the perfect car. He saved his money and bought a Ferrari. Then the car got a scratch; his response was to write a suicide note, stating, "There is nothing to live for," and therefore shot himself. For almost all, the scratch appears, to use a popular expression, to be small stuff, but not for him. His belief was "People with a scratch on a Ferrari ought to be dead." His logic can be symbolized by the following.

> People with a scratch on a Ferrari ought to be dead.
> I am a person who has a scratch on his Ferrari.
> *Therefore*, I ought to be dead.

Another Shneidman example is the elderly woman who killed herself after her canary died. Her cognition was, "People with a dead canary ought to be dead." She had her "*therefore.*" Thus, we must remember that trauma for both these individuals—and all suicidal people—was a perception, not "objective" reality. They are so blinded. They had their major premise and *the* trauma; he about a scratch on a car and she about a dead pet. What was the officer's trauma(s)? It is, however, so much more. It is not only simply about sinning or having a scratch on a car. It is not only simply about a demotion or a dead pet. It is not simply about losing a loved one. ("People rejected by Sam ought to be dead.")

Figuratively speaking, the suicidal person is intoxicated by overpowering emotions. Concomitantly, there is a constricted logic and perception. Although the person defines the trauma (situation), one cannot buy into the overpowering emotions and constricted logic presented by the individual, even in a retrospective investigation, a psychological autopsy or police investigation. Yet many do so after events like homicide-suicide.

One of the basics of a suicidal mind is the following: There is poverty of thought, exhibited by focusing only on permutations and combinations of grief and grief-provoking topics. A common premise is that something is either black or white. Something is either "A or not A." To presume that the suicidal individual either wants to kill himself or not is an extremely limited point of view, even if the person generates *only* such permutations and combinations in his premises. It is not necessary to require a view of the world as "A or not A" (e.g., Sam or no Sam, canary or no canary), that is, a view (or belief) of the world exhibiting only permutations and combinations of one content. The individual may only think of grief-provoking content, but he can also have other fantasies or cognitions. To suggest such an "A and not A" world is a limited and harsh view of life, one which neither the suicidal person nor we have to accept. Thus, the task is to not accept the first premise; and therefore, not the "therefore." We are not limited by what any suicidal person says, writes, communicates, believes, and so on. We, in fact, need to not buy into the suicidal person's (or homicidal person's) beliefs/cognitions; some of them may well be intentioned to mask the truth, reality, and so on.

Theory, explicit and implicit, like that presented, plays a key role in understanding any behavior (and for suicidal or homicidal-suicidal behavior, it is essential) (Leenaars, 2004). It is only through theory that we will sort out the booming buzzing confusion (mess) of suicide experience. We do not have to accept the mess. Perception is in the eye of the beholder (Kuhn, 1962). Yet do we accept the theory of the killer? The abandoned person? The man with the scratched Ferrari? The officer who received a demotion? The officer who was to be cuffed and jailed? Thus, it would be wise to reflect on the death officer's conclusion, her "therefore." We think many of us can be relatively sure—no, absolutely sure—that at least the scratch on the Ferrari is not cause to therefore kill oneself. Nor were Desdemona's. It is not cause to therefore kill someone else too, say the person who put the scratch on the car.

DISSEMBLING: CLUES TO SUICIDE RECONSIDERED

"Suicide happens without warning." This is a myth that Shneidman challenged (see earlier discussion, Suicide Facts and Myths). He stated that the fact was "Studies reveal that the suicidal person gives many clues and warnings regarding suicidal intentions." Another fact, according to Shneidman, was "Of 10 persons who kill themselves, 8 have given definite warnings of their suicidal intentions." However, is "Suicide happens without warning" really a fable? People, in fact, today believe that "Suicide happens without warning" is a myth (Leenaars et al., 1988). Yet forensically and clinically, the concern is if 8 out of 10 people give warnings, what about the other two? Officers are more concerned about this group too, such as in a suicide by cop situation. Goldblatt (1992) and Litman (1994) have separately noted that a small but noted percentage of completed suicides are seen as having left no clues. A minority of these people are most perplexing to even the most veteran forensic suicidologist. How do we understand and predict their suicide (Leenaars, 1997)?

The classical case, albeit a literary one, is Edwin Arlington Robinson's *Richard Cory* (1953). The poem describes Richard Cory as a "gentleman from sole to crown." He was "human, rich, favored, schooled," and, in fact, people "thought that he was everything." Then, as the poem ends, Richard Cory, unexpectedly puts a "bullet through his head." Here is Robinson's (1953) classical poem, one that many of us read in English class in high school:

Richard Cory
Whenever Richard Cory went down town,
We people on the pavement looked at him:
He was a gentleman from sole to crown,
Clean favored, and imperially slim.
And he was always quietly arrayed,
And he was always human when he talked;
But still he fluttered pulses when he said,
"Good-morning," and he glittered when he walked.
And he was rich—yes, richer than a king
And admirably schooled in every grace:
In fine, we thought that he was everything
To make us wish that we were in his place.
So on we worked, and waited for the light,
And went without the meat, and cursed the bread;
And Richard Cory, one calm summer night,
Went home and put a bullet through his head.

That suicide happened without warning. Did Othello's? The Richard Cory-type of patient is, in fact, a person whom many of us experience in our career. Bongar and Greaney (1994) in their studies, have found that the odds are greater than 50% of psychiatrists, and greater than 20% of psychologists losing a patient to suicide over the course of their careers. A patient committing suicide is, thus, not a rare event (Bongar, 1991), although the Richard Cory patient is not all of them. The fact is that over 80% of the people who killed themselves did leave clues. The other 20% raise our anxiety, with the Richard Cory-type being even more infrequent, but maybe not in police officers. A much publicized Canadian case was that of Dr. Suzanne Killinger Johnson, who in August 2000, jumped to her death with her infant at a subway station in Toronto. She was a clinician herself, who managed to hide her spiraling (dissembling) depression from her medically trained family. She was discussed on the front page of Canada's national newspaper, the *Globe and Mail*, over and over, and in every other media. She was what we call a Richard Cory-type of suicide. We need to understand the Richard Cory-type officer better.

In the 1990s, Shneidman (1994) had reconsidered his perspective on clues to suicide. He asked, "How it is that some people who are on the verge of suicide . . . can hide or mask their secretly held intentions?" Shneidman suggests that many clues are veiled, clouded, and guarded, some even misleading. He argues that there are individuals who live secret lives. These people do not communicate. They often lie. On the Rorschach, as an example for clinicians, they would score a high Lambda (Exner, 1986). These people do not process or mediate the stimuli in the usual way, having a defensive intent, conscious or unconscious, to avoid the situation. There are walls, whether blue, white, or otherwise. Often these walls reflect a basic coping style, with conscious and unconscious elements in the process (Leenaars & Lester, 1996a). Shneidman calls it *dissembling*.

Of course, the concept is not new; Shakespeare, for example, used the concept in *Othello*. In that play, Othello believes his beloved wife, Desdemona, is unfaithful. Othello rages inside and has a murderous plan; yet he masks, projecting a self-reflective statement on his wife. He dissembles so. Shakespeare writes,

> *Othello.* Well my good lady. [Aside]. O, hardness to dissemble.

Othello then kills his wife and to escape, he kills himself.

To dissemble means to conceal one's motives. It is to disguise or conceal one's feelings, intention, or even suicide risk. These people wear "masks." It is a masking. The story that they tell is that they *do not* tell their story; indeed, they themselves may be unaware of the dissembling or masking. There is frequently an enduring personality pattern. It is an enduring pattern of inner experience and behavior. For example, from an early age, they lie about everything, both omissions and commissions. The behavior often deviates markedly from the expectations of family, friends, and even of one's culture—or the culture of a group (or subculture), such as being a police officer (or is it?). Often, unconscious processes are involved. Kurt Cobain dissembled; he stated in his note that he is, "faking it and pretending as if I'm having 100% fun." Most police officers, border-security officers, clinicians, and the like, encounter such people, not only suicidal people, and not only homicidal people. Their stories are invalid; sometimes they even intentionally produce or feign a behavior (or symptom). Shneidman (1994) stated,

> We suicidologists who deal with potentially suicidal people must . . . understand that in the ambivalent flow and flux of life, some desperately suicidal people . . . can dissemble and hide their true lethal feelings from the world. (p. 395)

We *a priori* believe that this is especially important to remember about officers who die by suicide. They often dissemble with fellow officers, parents, girl/boyfriend, therapist, everyone. No one often predicts risk. The question raised, "Why?" (see below, Police Suicide, Classic and Current).

A PERSPECTIVE ON THE PSYCHOLOGICAL AUTOPSY

It is now well accepted that the specific procedure within forensic suicidology that would assist in investigating/studying an officer's suicide or homicide-suicide is called the *psychological autopsy* (Seltzer, Croktan, & Bartholomew, 2001). The psychological autopsy may include the following questions: Why did the individual kill himself? How did the individual die and when; that is, why at a particular time? and, Although already established in many cases, what is the most probable mode of death? Yet the latter question does occur.

In the psychological autopsy, data are obtained through interviews with survivors, persons close to the deceased, including, for example, family, friends, doctors, and fellow officers. Facts and circumstances from newspapers, historical records (e.g. school), anatomical autopsies, suicide notes, Internet writing, personnel records, medical/mental health records, and police records are obtained and other procedures are utilized. It is on this basis that one can begin to answer the above questions and, specifically here: Why did Lt. Michael Pigott kill himself?

How is the psychological autopsy conducted? As this is the work of the authors' mentor, Edwin Shneidman, we will here quote him from the author's edited volume of Shneidman's selected works, *Lives and Deaths* (1999a):

> How is a psychological autopsy performed? Talking to some key persons—spouse, lover, parent, grown child, friend, colleague, physician, supervisor, and co-worker—who knew the decedent, does it. The talking to is done gently, a mixture of conversation, interview, emotional support, general questions, and a good deal of listening. I always telephone and then go out to the home. After rapport is established, a good general opening question might be: "Please tell me, what was he (she) like?" Sometimes clothes and material possessions are looked at, photographs shown, and even diaries and correspondence shared. (On one occasion, the widow showed me her late husband's suicide note—which she had hidden from the police!—rather changing the equivocal nature of the death.)
>
> In general, I do not have a fixed outline in mind while conducting a psychological autopsy, but inasmuch as outlines have been requested from time to time, one is presented below with the dual cautions that it should not be followed slavishly and that the investigator should be ever mindful that he may be asking questions that are very painful to people in an obvious grief-laden situation. The person who conducts a psychological autopsy should participate, as far as he is genuinely able, in the anguish of the bereaved person and should always do his work with the mental health of the survivors in mind.
>
> Here, then, are some categories that might be included in a psychological autopsy (Shneidman, 1977):
>
> 1. Information identifying victim (name, age, address, marital status, religious practices, occupation, and other details)
> 2. Details of the death (including the cause or method and other pertinent details)
> 3. Brief outline of victim's history (siblings, marriage, medical illness, medical treatment, psychotherapy, suicide attempts)
> 4. Death history of victim's family (suicides, cancer, other fatal illnesses, ages of death, and other details)
> 5. Description of the personality and life-style of the victim

6. Victim's typical patterns of reaction to stress, emotional upsets, and periods of disequilibrium
7. Any recent—from last few days to last twelve months—upsets, pressures, tensions, or anticipations of trouble
8. Role of alcohol or drugs in (a) overall life-style of victim, and (b) his death. *(We would add questions, given the police cases, about guns)*
9. Nature of victim's interpersonal relationships (including those with physicians)
10. Fantasies, dreams, thoughts, premonitions, or fear of victim relating to death, accident, or suicide
11. *Changes* in the victim before death (of habits, hobbies, eating, sexual patterns, and other life routines)
12. Information relating to the "life side" of victim (up-swings, successes, plans)
13. Assessment of intention, that is, role of the victim in his own demise
14. Rating of lethality
15. Reaction of informants to victim's death
16. Comments, special features, and so on.

In conducting the interviews during a psychological autopsy, it is often best to ask open-ended questions that permit the respondent to associate to relevant details without being made painfully aware of the specific interests of the questioner. As an example: I might be very interested in knowing whether or not there was a change (specifically, a recent sharp decline) in the decedent's eating habits. Rather than ask directly, "Did his appetite drop recently?" a question almost calculated to elicit a defensive response, I have asked a more general question such as, "Did he have any favourite foods?" Obviously, my interest is not to learn what foods he preferred. Not atypically, the respondent will tell me what the decedent's favourite foods were and then go on to talk about recent changes in his eating habits—"Nothing I fixed for him seemed to please him"—and even proceed to relate other recent changes, such as changing patterns in social or sexual or recreational habits, changes which diagnostically would seem to be related to a dysphoric person, not inconsistent with a suicidal or subintentioned death. (Leenaars, 1999a, pp. 399–400)

A POLICE PERSPECTIVE ON THE PSYCHOLOGICAL AUTOPSY

Robert Loo (2001), a well-respected expert on police suicide and former RCMP psychologist, offers some insights on the psychology autopsies, with special reference to the police. We here quote verbatim:

By changing to a multidisciplinary approach, the Death Investigation Team, involving behavioral scientists in addition to the traditional medical experts, greater success resulted in (psychological) autopsies. In addition, the interviewing of informants such as family members, friends, family physician, and

> co-workers added much independent information about the suicided and circumstances (Brent, 1989).

Since that time the term and process has evolved and broadened in scope; we are concerned only about the psychological autopsy in the context of police suicide. For us, psychological autopsies are useful in addressing three broad questions.

What was the Mode of Suicide?

Seeing as the majority of police who suicide use their service handgun, the method of suicide is usually easy to confirm. In some cases, such as hanging, asphyxiation (e.g., carbon monoxide poisoning from vehicle exhaust), or drug overdose, the mode of suicide can also be easily confirmed. On the other hand, some cases can be more difficult to resolve because they involve multiple methods; for example, a drug overdose and drowning in a bathtub. Even more difficult to resolve are suicides that may appear as accidental deaths. For example, the single-vehicle fatal accident where an officer drives at high speed into a solid barrier when there are no mechanical, road, or weather conditions that can be proposed as reasonable explanations for the apparent suicide.

There are several main reasons for gathering these data. The obvious reason is to identify use of the service handgun or other departmental weapon such as a shotgun so that access might be better controlled, hopefully, to make future suicides using departmental firearms more difficult.

What were the Circumstances Surrounding the Suicide?

Determining when and where suicides occur might have implications for prevention (Lester, 1987).

- Did the suicide occur on or off duty?
- Did the suicide occur on a weekday, weekend, or holiday?
- Did the suicide occur at night or during the day?
- Did the suicide occur at home, a police facility, patrol vehicle, or other notable location?
- Did the suicide occur on an anniversary or other special day?
- Did the officer give away personal effects just prior to the suicide or make other gestures suggesting a farewell, a settling of accounts, or reconciliation with others?
- Was there a noticeable mood change before the suicide?
- Was alcohol or drugs a factor at the time of the suicide?

These data could identify patterns suggesting periods when managers and helpers need to be especially vigilant about potential suicides so that preventive actions could be taken. For example, if mood changes precede suicide, then supervisors and officers should be trained to identify such changes to help identify high-risk officers.

Why Did the Officer Commit Suicide?

This is a critical question not only for identifying prevention actions but it is a question raised by survivors who might benefit, in a small way, from having the answer. Family, friends, and fellow officers raise this question, wondering what could have been so disturbing in the officer's life that suicide was the way out. For many officers, suicide follows not just a single problem or critical event but the culmination of several overwhelming problems such as combined marital problems and career frustrations.

Ethical Issues

In conducting a psychological autopsy, one must treat all information and documentation as confidential. The integrity of the deceased must be respected. One must be careful not to cause further distress to survivors, for example, in the interview process. It is preferable that health professionals who are governed by a code of ethical conduct and subjected to disciplinary action by their professional body conduct interviews of survivors and informants. In any case, all members of the team conducting the psychological autopsy need to be selected for their related expertise and personal suitability (Loo, 2001, unnumbered).

RES IPSA LOQUITUR

Following Shneidman's lead (see Shneidman, 1977), reports should follow the principle of *res ipsa loquitur:* The facts speak for themselves. The documents, newspaper accounts, letters, investigation reports, third-party interviews, clinical records, and so on speak for themselves. This is the principle for the psychology autopsy, and we follow such in the book, beginning with the case below of Vince Foster Jr.

CASE ILLUSTRATION: VINCENT FOSTER JR.

Our attempt to address the question, "Why do people kill themselves?" has, we hope, brought us closer to an answer. We now see that suicide, indeed, can be best understood as a multidimensional event. It is constituted, at least, by intrapsychic aspects (unbearable pain, cognitive constriction, indirect expressions, inability to adjust, vulnerable ego) and interpersonal aspects (interpersonal relations, rejection-aggression, identification-egression). Suicide has adjustive value for the individual, not survival value (Murray, 1967). It is perceived, consciously and unconsciously, as the best solution to a problem. It is an escape.

In support of Shneidman (1985), there are more psychological commonalities than differences in suicidal people. There are commonalities across age, sex, culture, time, occupation, and method chosen for suicide (and maybe other factors in suicidal people). Yet good theory in suicidology also has to have sound clinical and forensic utility. We will briefly address the applicability of the presented schema by examining the application of the theory to the case illustration of Vince Foster Jr.

To return to the "trunk" of suicide, which is the current basis of "best practice" understanding, let us present a case: Vincent Foster Jr. Case presentations have an important place in suicidology (Allport, 1942, 1962), and despite limitations, the person is the main business of our everyday work. Vince Foster Jr. was President Bill Clinton's deputy White House counsel, who shot himself with his father's gun on July 20, 1993. Vincent Foster was Clinton's friend. He was 48, married, and had three children. Foster had been in Washington for 6 months when he was found dead in a park on the northern Virginia side of the Potomac River. Here is his suicide note:

> I made mistakes from ignorance, inexperience and overwork
>
> I did not knowingly violate any law or standard of conduct
>
> No one in the White House, to my knowledge, violated any law or standard of conduct, including any action in the travel office.
>
> The FBI lied in their report to the AG [attorney general]
>
> The Press is covering up the illegal benefits they received from the travel staff
>
> The GOP has lied and misrepresented its knowledge and role and covered up a prior investigation
>
> The Ushers Office plotted to have excessive costs incurred, taking advantage of Khaki [White House Designer] and HRC [Hilary Rodham Clinton]
>
> The public will never believe the innocence of the Clintons and their loyal staff
>
> The WSJ [Wall Street Journal] editors lie without consequence
>
> I was not meant for the job or the spotlight of public life in Washington. Here ruining people is considered sport.

What can we learn from Vincent Foster Jr.'s note? Utilizing the model outlined, we learn the following hypotheses:

1. Unbearable Psychological Pain—Vincent Foster's mind, based on the note, was permeated with pain—the pain of pain. The suicide was seen as an escape. Although there were likely many motives, the accusations by the FBI, press, GOP, and so on, of violating the law or standards of misconduct overwhelmed him. Mr. Foster was forlorn and distressed. He could not endure nor cope with the injustices, feeling so hopeless and helpless.

2. Cognitive Constriction—Vincent Foster's mind was a constricted mind. He was "intoxicated" with the trauma—"ruining people is considered sport." His note is only permutations of that trauma.
3. Indirect Expressions—Vincent Foster Jr. was overwhelmingly angry. Yet the anger became turned inward. Indeed, it is quite clear that the manifest aspects of his note imply much more latently. One must speculate on unconscious dynamics as the driving force to his death.
4. Inability to Adjust—Vincent Foster could not cope; he saw himself as too weak to adjust to "the spotlight of public life in Washington." He is, in fact, so passionate in his reverie of that topic. Indeed, his state of mind was indicative of a mental disorder. Vincent Foster likely suffered from, at least, a depressive disorder.
5. Ego—Vincent Foster's ego was weakened; he lacked constructive tendencies. There is such pain over his unresolved problem—the accusations. He feels so punished.
6. Interpersonal relations—Mr. Foster was weakened and defeated by the FBI, the Wall Street Journal, and even the public. Indeed, Vincent Foster lists a long history, experiencing the world as traumatic. Vince Foster committed suicide because of a frustration of needs—these included attachment, affiliation (the White House), autonomy, defendance (to defend), harm avoidance, and infavoidance (to avoid humiliation). (Murray, 1938).
7. Rejection-Aggression—Vince Foster felt so rejected. Indeed, the rejection was a narcissistic injury—narcissism, of course, is central to this type of executive suicide. Vince Foster, and individuals like him, struggle against narcissistic catastrophes. Foster is so angry but so weakened by the lies of the press, the GOP, and the public. Indeed, he is so weakened that he turns the aggressive impulses against himself. He kills himself, although his suicide, especially the note, was calculatedly written to have an impact on the press, the FBI, and so on. Vince Foster wanted revenge.
8. Identification-Egression—Vincent Foster Jr. was so attached to the Clintons, the White House, law, and standards of conduct. These were deep ideals and identifications. With the loss of these attachments (ideals), he needed to escape, egress. Death became the *only* solution.

[The actual protocol sentences (see Table 2, TGSP) that were verified in Foster's note are as follows: Unbearable Pain: 1, 2, 3, 4, 5, 6; Cognitive Constriction: 7, 8, 9; Indirect Expressions: 11, 12—no ambivalence (10); Inability to Adjust: 13, 14, 15; Ego: 16, 17, 18; Interpersonal Relations: 19, 20, 21, 22; Rejection-Aggression: 25, 26 (narcissism), 27, 30, 31, 32; Identification-Egression: 33, 34, 35.]

Can we learn more? Fortunately, because of Mr. Foster's relationship to then-President Clinton, a psychological autopsy was undertaken and a brief synopsis appeared in Maris, Berman, and Silverman (2000). This autopsy allows us to place the note and its analysis within the larger context of Foster's life (We borrow here from records, keeping in mind that the note and above analysis was undertaken well before the psychological autopsy was presented). One can see how the analyzed note is mirrored in the psychological autopsy.

Vincent Foster Jr.'s life was described as one of "success and distinction." This included president of his high school class, first in his law class, top score on Arkansas bar exam, partner of a top law firm, and so on. He was listed in "Best Lawyers in America." He was a success and had a reputation of high standards, something quite obvious in his note.

Vincent Foster Jr. was narcissistically attached to his ideals, law, and standards of conduct. One's reputation was everything—he needed to be first in his class. Public self *was* self. He spoke a few months before his death about one's public image at the University of Arkansas Law School:

> The reputation you develop for intellectual and ethical integrity will be your greatest asset or your worst enemy. You will be judged by your judgment. Treat every pleading, every brief, every contract, every letter, every daily task as if your career will be judged on it.

Those statements made the note and his death more understandable. Days after his speech at the law school, the accusations by the FBI, the press, GOP, and so on, began. "Travelgate" occurred; he began to be judged about financial misuse of travel, the use of the FBI, and so on. The Wall Street Journal even questioned his public behavior, and on June 17th wrote an editorial "Who is Vincent Foster?" A narcissistic injury occurred. Vincent Foster Jr. had been described as "The Rock of Gibraltar," and then in Washington, he was defeated. He is said to have been disgraced. He became "intoxicated" with the loss of his ideals. In his presentation at the law school, he had said, "Dents to reputations are irreparable." There was a dent, an unbearable pain. He became forlorn and distressed. Foster looked "blue," "down," "out of it," and "frustrated" (e.g., his needs, i.e., infavoidance, (Perhaps a brief definition of "infavoidance," as this is the first instance of its use.) were frustrated). Foster, in his constricted mind, even believed that he was a liability—a dent—to President Clinton. Vincent could not cope. He, as the note reveals, was depressed. He could not cope—a man who always got A's, got an F. Death became the only solution—as noted in the psychological autopsy, he could not return to Arkansas. Suicide became the only solution.

Yet his life, like the note, reveals unconscious dynamics. For example, what does it mean to use his father's gun—a 1913 Colt Army service revolver? Did Foster feel a dent or as he said, "a blemish on (his) reputation?" And his family, what more could we learn? And President Clinton, what did Clinton mean to Foster? Did Foster see a dent in President Clinton, who we later learned suffered in his public reputation in the Monica Lewinsky affair? The notes, like his psychological autopsy, reveal much—but does it say it all? And could we, aspiring to rescue, have saved Foster? Would psychotherapy have helped? Medication? Hospitalization? Controlling the environment? And what about the fellow officer?

PREVENTION/INTERVENTION/POSTVENTION

The classical approach to prevention, whether mental health or public health, is that of Caplan (1964), who differentiated between primary, secondary, and tertiary prevention. The more commonly used concepts today for these three modes of *prevention* in suicidology are prevention, intervention, and postvention, respectively. Caplan's view still provides a sound model for a response to suicide at any of the possible levels, from individual to society (and will have application to the recommendations made from the studies). Briefly, the three modes of a comprehensive response to a person at risk are as follows:

Prevention relates to the principle of good mental hygiene in general. It consists of strategies to ameliorate the conditions that lead to suicide—to do something before the event occurs. Preventing suicide is best accomplished through primary prevention, primarily by education. Officers must be educated about suicide, about homicide and domestic violence. Such education—given that suicide is a multidimensional event—is enormously complicated. Be that as it may, there are numerous suicide (primary) prevention programs available in police services in the United States, Canada, and around the world.

Intervention relates to the treatment and care of a suicidal crisis or suicidal problem. Secondary prevention is doing something during the event. Suicide is a multidimensional event, and thus, is not solely a medical problem, and many people can serve as lifesaving agents. Nonetheless, professionally trained people, psychologists, psychiatrists, social workers, psychiatric nurses, crisis workers, and so on continue to play the primary roles in intervention, and the psychologists/psychiatrists with police services belonging to this list. Thus, although equally true for prevention and postvention, intervention will call for the development of community and social linkages, a hallmark of an evidence-based response to intervention. There is a lot that any community can do.

Postvention, a term introduced by Shneidman (1973, 1975), refers to those things done after the event has occurred. Postvention deals with the traumatic aftereffects in the survivors of a person who has committed suicide (or in those close to someone who has attempted suicide). There were/are many survivors. Postvention in suicide or homicide-suicide involves offering mental health and public health services to the bereaved survivors. Family, friends, police officers, local service providers, and so on, need help in the loss and grief. Postvention includes working with all survivors who are in need. Of course, as is well established (Shneidman, 1985), psychological autopsies are effective postvention and often help in the healing.

CONCLUDING REMARKS

People in general have considerable difficulty appreciating significant characteristics of suicidal individuals. Most fortunately, a host of suicidologists have given us a rich history of theory for understanding suicide. These suicidologists point out that the suicidal history is understandable and thus, predictable and controllable.

The main conclusion is that there may be more commonalities (agreement or sameness) in suicide than differences. By virtue of our human quality, whether male or female, whether police officer or not, greater similarities than differences are to be expected in all suicidal events (Shneidman, 1991). Maybe there are forms, seals, archetypes, unity thema, commonalities, or whatever we wish to call *it*. We presented an array of commonalities. Despite clear and distinct commonalities, each individual must still be, however, understood idiosyncratically (uniquely), even if dissembling. This is so in police.

We need to continue to develop multidimensional models (Goffman, 1974; Kuhn, 1962) to understand suicide—and the suicide of that individual, whether Vincent Foster Jr. or any police suicide, that can be researched, and most importantly, can be made useful and life saving. What would have helped with Vincent? What intervention (psychotherapy, healing circle, medication, hospitalization, and so on) will effectively work with that individual? We need to be evidence-based. What empirically supported recommendations can be made that are effective with that suicidal police officer? Suicidal people? We need to be person centered (or oriented)—what kind of person that person is. This is true for clinicians, police officers, community-based individuals, clergy, Elders, survivors—all who work at suicide prevention. It is true for us who are bent on changing the lifelong adjustment patterns of the suicidal person, not only to help rescue the person today, but also to assist for the future. We want to change the deadly "sameness." The goal of our book is simple: to help the suicidal person cope with life. What recommendations can be made? What can we learn from police officers who died by suicide? What can we learn from police who kill and commit suicide?

What could we have done to help? Could Vincent's suicide have been stopped? Could Kelly's homicide-suicide have been stopped? Would psychotherapy have helped? Medication? There was so much pain and anguish, a psychache in Vincent's life. What would have worked to prevent the officer's death? And why did his fellow officer survive his pain, and his partner not? What were the fellow officer's protective factors? Why did *that officer* die and his father, her ex-husband, his friends, her fellow officers and so on, survive? These are the most important (individual) questions. These are some of the questions one asks in psychological autopsies. Why did Vincent Foster Jr., or as we will learn later, Chief Thomas Moffatt jump into death? And what could we have done to prevent these needless deaths?

In Herman Melville's—who was an equally troubled soul—monumental study of people's anguish and suicide, *Moby Dick*, Chapter 36, "The Quarter Deck," Captain Ahab, an Othello-type person, speaks:

> Hark ye yet again—the little lower layer. All visible objects, man, are but as pasteboard masks. But in each event—in the living act, the undoubted deed—there some unknown but still reasoning thing puts forth the mouldings of its features from behind the unreasoning mask. If man will strike, strike through the mask! How can the prisoner reach outside except by thrusting through the wall.

We—police officers, clinicians, survivors, and so on—must understand and reach through the suicidal mask.

CHAPTER 2

Homicide. Suicide: Are They Related?

This chapter asks a main question of this volume: Are homicide and suicide related?

Death is superordinate to suicide. Suicide is one category of the four universally recognized modes of death: natural, accident, suicide, and homicide—what Shneidman called the NASH categories of death. Of course, some notions of death are always involved in the suicidal and homicidal scenario. It makes sense, thus, for a suicidologist to study the topic of homicide. Sigmund Freud did so, as do the forensic homicidologists: Nancy Allen, Enrico Ferri, Andrew Henry and James Short. They all believe that suicide and homicide is a stream of violence, not that distinct from each other.

Almost a million people die by suicide worldwide each year. Over a half a million die by homicide. It is not known how many die by homicide-suicide. These numbers are enormous, never mind the multitude of survivors. No single factor or event explains why so many people are violent. Suicide and homicide are multidetermined. They are the result of an interplay of individual, relationship, social, cultural, and environmental factors. This is sometimes called the ecological model. The model has been applied to a vast array of behaviors, most recently violence, including self-directed violence (WHO, 2002), and we do so in this book.

Suicide is violence. Homicide is violence. Suicide is self-directed violence. Homicide is other-directed violence. They are lethal violence. Suicide, homicide, and other violence have probably always been part of the human experience. There are many possible ways of defining suicide and homicide.

We defined suicide in Chapter 1. How can we define homicide? We will explore some facts in this chapter.

This chapter answers at least the following questions: Are suicide and homicide related? How are they associated? How can we understand homicide and suicide, and together? Is suicide by cop related? We will show that suicide and homicide together is, indeed, a *stream*. In the next chapters we will explain

http://dx.doi.org/10.2190/SHSC2

suicide among police, both classical and current studies, and homicide-suicide, including in police.

* * * * * *

INTRODUCTION

Suicide is violence. Homicide is violence. Suicide is self-directed violence. Homicide is other-directed violence. They are lethal violence. Suicide, homicide and other violence have probably always been part of the human experience. There are many possible ways of defining violence. The World Health Organization (WHO, 2002) defines violence as

> The intentional use of physical force or power, threatened or actual, against oneself, another person, or against a group or community, that either results in or has a high likelihood of resulting in injury, death, psychological harm, maldevelopment or deprivation. (p. 5)

Intentionality is central; one of the more complex aspects of the definition is the matter of intentionality. It was central to the definition of suicide (see Chapter 1 and below). The Oxford English Dictionary (OED) defines intentional as "done on purpose." Intentionality is the noun. It is to have as one's purpose. It is a conscious act. One intends suicide. One has a purpose—to be dead, self-induced annihilation. Homicide is the same; it is other-induced annihilation.

In Chapter 1, we defined suicide as

> Currently in the Western world, suicide is a conscious act of self-induced annihilation, best understood as a multidimensional event in a needful individual who defines an issue for which the suicide is perceived as the best solution.

If that is so, we can define homicide as

> Currently in the Western world, homicide is a conscious act of other-induced annihilation, best understood as a multidimensional event in a needful individual who defines an issue for which the homicide is perceived as the best solution.

It is estimated that 1.6 million people die by violence each year. Almost half (800,000) of these are suicides; one third are homicides (530,000) and one-fifth (320,000) are war related. This is an enormous, never mind the survivors, cost of violence. No single factor or event explains why so many people are violent. Violence is multidetermined. Suicide, homicide, and the like is the result of an interplay of individual, relationship, social, cultural, and environmental factors. This is sometimes called the ecological model (Bronfenbrenner, 1979; Dahlberg & Krug, 2002; Jenkins & Singh, 2000). First applied to child abuse (Garbarino & Crouter, 1978), the model has been applied to a vast array of behaviors, most recently violence, including self-directed violence (WHO, 2002) (see Figure 1).

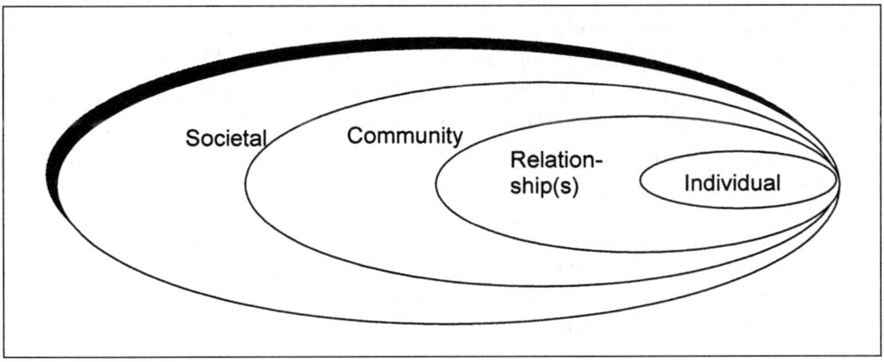

Figure 1. Ecological model for understanding suicide.

The model simply suggests that there are different levels, that is, individual, relationship, community, and societal, which influence suicide and homicide, and thus, by implication, one can address behavior at various levels. Comprehensive (ecological) approaches target not only the individual but also the factors beyond the individual. These approaches are also focused on the relationship (e.g., family members, relations with fellow officers), community, and societal levels.

CULTURE: A FEW THOUGHTS

Before we turn to the question posed, we want to raise some *a priori* questions about culture. Culture is figural in the ecological model. First, of course, what is it that we are talking about? What is culture? What is blue culture? What are we referring to with the word "culture group?" This is a first step. What are we studying in this volume, when we state "police" in our title? The *Oxford English Dictionary* (OED) defines culture as:

> **4** The cultivation or development of the mind, manners, etc.; improvement by education and training. E16. **5** Refinement of mind, tastes, and manners; artistic and intellectual development; the artistic and intellectual side of civilization. E19. **6** A particular form, stage, or type of intellectual development or civilization in a society; a society or group characterized by its distinctive customs, achievements, products, outlook, etc. M19. **7** The distinctive customs, achievements, products, outlook, etc., of a society or group; the way of life of a society or group.

Although this explanation falls short, it provides at least a first attempt at definition. It suggests that culture is a cultivation and this *results* in a community or society having shared skills and knowledge, shared ways of doing things—even in suicide. This would be true for police. They are a community. Culture is a collective meaning: to allow people to know who they are, where they come from, and where they are going—again, even in suicide. This is also true for police. This is entirely consistent with Leong and Leach's (2008) definition of culture as *worldview*. Police have a worldview. One of the best definitions of culture that we have ever read is from *The Royal Commission on Aboriginal Peoples* (1995) in Canada; they wrote,

> Culture is the whole complex of relationships, knowledge, languages, social institutions, beliefs, values and ethical rules that bind a people together and give a collective and its individual members a sense of who they are and where they belong. (p. 25)

Culture is rooted in one's people, whether from a society such as the United States or Canada or a group such as a police service. Culture is one's meaning, who you are and where you belong—even in death (Leenaars, 2009a; Leenaars, Maris, & Takahashi, 1997; Leong & Leach, 2008;). As we stated some years ago, "The individual—such as John—is among other things a social being. Individuals live in a meaningful world. Culture may well give us meaning in the world. It may well give the world its theories/perspectives" (Leenaars, Maris, & Takahashi, 1997, p. 2).

Although we do not think that culture will ever be clearly and distinctly defined, at least the definitions offered allow us to know better what we are talking about. What are we talking about when we write police culture, or more commonly referred to as blue culture (Danto, 1978; Rudofossi, 2007). This means that by the very fact of being from a different group or community or society or even nation, we are different. We are our culture. Police are their own blue culture. Specific examples of the blue culture are to adhere to the macho outlook or tradition and to take great pride in the achievement of possessing a service gun. This raises, thus, a number of questions on our topic of suicide and homicide: Is suicide the same? Or is it different? What about homicide? Are people from a police service in the United States so different from other Americans when they kill themselves? Are there commonalities? Or are there factors or aspects that are different, such as specific blue aspects? How can we study suicide in different communities, such as the police? Can we apply our understanding of suicide and homicide to all people? To only police groups? If we need to change our theory with police, what do we need to change? Do we need to change at the individual or relationship(s) or community or society levels? What are they? Can being a member of a police group contribute to suicide? Are there barriers or walls to wellness, often called blue walls? And, after we have answered these questions, there are many more, not only in study but in praxis. What blue culturally sensitive interventions are needed? What policies and procedures are needed to be sensitive to, but not enable, blue walls? Is some if it suicidogenic, or even homicidogenic? Having raised such questions, we hope the reader will think beyond the individual officer and think about the relationship(s), social, cultural, and environmental factors too. You need to know the blue culture, among many other factors or aspects, to know the officer and his suicide or homicide-suicide.

SUICIDE AND HOMICIDE

According to the WHO (2002), "While some risk factors may be unique to particular types of violence, the various types of violence more commonly share a number of risk factors" (pp. 13–14). There are associations between suicide and several other types of violence, especially homicide (Allen, 1980, 1993; Malmquist, 1996; Stevenson & Cox, 2008; WHO, 2002). They are associated in multifaceted ways, and by implication, because violence is a multifaceted problem with biological, psychological, social, and environmental factors, it needs to be confronted on several different levels at once. The ecological model guides us. And, on one more point, from the model's implications, violence is largely preventable (WHO, 2002, 2006). However, to do so, a comprehensive prevention approach is needed.

Yet the questions can be posed: Are suicide and homicide related? How are they associated? How can we understand homicide and suicide among police?

The public typically distinguishes between homicide and suicide. They are seen as fundamentally different. Indeed, even police, professionals, coroners, politicians, the media, and so on distinguish between them. Yet there is a different way, as we are already hinting at, to understand the behavior. Homicide and suicide may be more similar than often believed. There are commonalities (or common factors).

In the Western world, suicide and homicide were not always seen as different. Early Christian thought made no distinction. St. Augustine categorically saw suicide and homicide as the same; like homicide, suicide violated the commandment, "Thou shalt not kill." Only God had power over man's life and death. Homicide and suicide were greater sins than any other. This was not only true for Christians, but also for many other religions; for example, Muslims, Hindus, and Buddhists. These views continue today. Suicide in the Western world, in fact, is a relatively new term, probably dating from the 1600s. Before that, the words used were self-killing or self-murder. The classical and current German term is in keeping with this tradition: *Selbstmord* or self-murder.

In science, Enrico Morselli (1882) and Enrico Ferri (1917) saw homicide-suicide as having the same underlying principle. This position was criticized by the well-known sociologist, Emile Durkheim (1897/1951). Sigmund Freud (1924/1974), however, held the same view as Ferri and Morselli. He saw suicide as homicide turned inward on the self (see Chapter 1). Freud (1924) noted,

> Just as the suicidal person may be attempting to kill an introjected ambivalently regarded other, the murderer may be killing an object of projection; the other, then is one in whom one sees one's own badness. The close linking of suicide and murder is seen in the mechanism of seeking to be killed, to be punished for one's own transgressions particularly for one's own murderous feelings. (as cited in Allen, 1980, pp. 86–88)

Of course, many other scientists hold to Freud's or Ferri's view. Yet it was probably Andrew Henry and James Short (1954) who constructed the best-known theoretical explanation of the relationship between homicide and suicide (Unnithan, Corzine, Huff-Corzine, & Whitt, 1994).

Of course, there are differences between homicide and suicide, but there is much to be gained by following Henry and Short. (Indeed, with homicide-suicide in police cases, we have no choice. We are, in fact, forced to do so.) Despite accepting unique differences, both general and specific, we need a unifying model, a best fit possible (not perfect) at this time. Unnithan et al. (1994) stated the basic argument as

> Although there are disagreements between homicide and suicide, there is much to be gained from revitalizing the theory developed by Henry and Short. Specifically, there are numerous issues related to lethal violence that can be better addressed—and, in some cases, understood—by working from an integrated model that emphasizes the similarities between self-directed and other-directed violence . . . . We are not, however, advocating a cessation of research that views homicide and suicide as distinct behaviours. Depending on the topic of investigation, this approach may be entirely appropriate and reasonable. Our contention is that for many research questions related to human violence, the goal of explanation will be better served by a theoretical model that explicitly takes into account the connections between homicide and suicide. (p. 5)

For any police case, we agree!

Suicide is self-induced annihilation. To understand suicide, as we have stated, it is useful to understand related topics of violence, especially homicide. In fact, suicide and homicide can be seen as interwoven expressions of the same stream, called the "stream analogy" of violence. Both can be conceptualized as a lethal response to frustration of needs, differing only in the direction in which the response is expressed.

The stream analogy of lethal violence is not new to this century. In the 1800s, two Italian scholars, Enrico Ferri and Enrico Morselli were best known for the idea. Their position was strongly criticized, however, by Emile Durkheim (1897/1951), who espoused that "suicide sometimes co-exists with homicide, sometimes they are mutually exclusive" (p. 355). In science, Copernicus was not the only great scientist silenced. For approximately a century, Durkheim's view dominated sociology and forensic study; Sigmund Freud in psychology, however, held to a view consistent with the stream analogy. In 1954, Henry and Short resurrected the view.

Historically, Ferri and Morselli noted that different social groups (or nations) had different rates of suicide and homicide and raised an important question. Why do persons in some social groups kill themselves more while other groups commit murders more? For example, why do Americans kill others more and themselves less compared with Canadians (Leenaars & Lester, 1994b)? Given their close geographic and cultural proximity, that fact is worth remembering by all officers and forensic specialists in those two nations. (There are many other differences in suicide and homicide in those two nations.) Thus, do not assume, around the world, that a suicide is a suicide or that a homicide-suicide is a homicide-suicide (Leenaars, 2007).

Unnithan et al. (1994), following Henry and Short, suggest that there is a stream of available destructiveness in a social group (or culture). Ferri called this production. They propose that this can be measured by what they call lethal violence rate (LVR). LVR measures the size of the stream of violence [LVR = Suicide (S) + Homicide (H)]. The direction of the stream, as Ferri called it, can be measured, on the other hand, by the suicide-murder ratio, SHR. SHR gauges the proportion of the total, which is expressed as suicide rather than homicide (SHR = S/(S + H).

Unnithan et al. suggest that these two measures allow one to understand the specific lethal violence in groups. From an integrated model, they write,

> At the individual level, both forms of lethal violence result from a combination of negative life events (frustration, stress) with attributional styles that locate blame either in the self (suicide) or in others (homicide). (p. 94)

Prediction is based, they argue, on attribution. Attribution is a product of situational and cultural factors. Ferri and Morselli had espoused biological factors (degeneration, impotence, or decay of the organism), whereas Unnithan et al., like Henry and Short, present a more social meaning view, and where Freud presented a more individual view (see ecological model).

Of course, this view is not without criticism. After Durkheim, Jack Douglas (1967) was most critical and influential. He wrote, "it is not possible to explain specific types of social events such as suicide in terms of abstract social meaning" (p. 339), nor could one of homicide-suicide. Moreover, Douglas maintained that the data on which statistical studies are based are inherently biased. However, more recent analysis suggests that one can, reliably, use mortality data. Indeed, it is a well-established fact that we need multiple sources to understand violence, for example, personal documents, third-party interviews, research on attempters (of suicide and homicide) and mortality statistics, something that we do in all police cases, in fact. There should be no single technique (or assessment); one must be multimodal in technique and approach in all police cases (Leenaars, 2004).

The importance of this model is that the stream analogy of violence resurfaces for the homicidologist-suicidologist, which is something that allows us to better understand annihilation, whether homicide or suicide, or homicide-suicide.

On a footnote, it can be asked whether this is true for males and females. The answer appears to be, yes (Johnson & Hotton, 2003; Leenaars, 2004).

On one further footnote, we highly encourage the reader to consult some classic texts on homicide. Space limits us here. At least, we recommend Nancy Allen's *Homicide* (1980, a person the author has consulted with on the topic on a number of occasions). Dr. Allen highly recommended Donald Lunde's *Murder and Madness* (1975).

To conclude, a question raised by David Lester (1987) on homicide and suicide was, Are they polar opposites? As we have seen, from an ecological view, murder is violence, and suicide is violence. They are intentional acts of aggression. Suicide is the human act of self-inflicted, self-intentional cessation. Homicide is the human act of other-inflicted, other-intentional cessation. Can homicide and suicide then be opposite behaviors? Scientifically, this is a difficult question as there have been few studies that have compared suicides and homicides (Lester, Perdue, & Brockhart, 1974).

Several types of suicidal and homicidal behaviors exist that appear to transcend the simple dichotomy. Homicide-suicide is the obvious one; and, as will be discussed below, it is not uncommon for murderers to commit suicide after murdering their victim (Allen, 1980, 1993; Lester, 1987). Yet many, such as Palermo et al. (1997) equally argue for homicide-suicide to be seen as separate from homicide. We believe a more comprehensive perspective is needed. There are several possible reasons for some killers killing themselves after the homicide, and we share below the insights from those studies. Police cases and research will illustrate the commonalities. In fact, Lester (1987) has concluded,

> All murderers are not alike. Megargee (1966) has distinguished between the overcontrolled murderer (who is calm, peaceable, and unaggressive much of the time, but who explodes occasionally into dramatically violent behavior) and the undercontrolled murderer (who is continually assaultive to the least frustration or insult). Clearly, these two kinds of murders handle their aggressive impulses very differently. Similarly, suicidal people differ. Some are chronically suicidal, making repeated suicide attempts before, in some cases, eventually killing themselves. Others who kill themselves have no history of prior suicidal behavior (Lester & Beck, 1976). These two types of suicidal individuals may be appropriately characterized as undercontrolled and overcontrolled, respectively. Identification of types of murderers and suicides may eventually lead to a better understanding of which factors (intrapsychic, interpersonal, and situational) lead some individuals to direct their aggression outwards while others turn aggression against themselves. (p. 59)

SUICIDE BY COP

Before we conclude, a tangent that can be raised is whether victim-precipitated homicide, or more specifically what is often called *suicide by cop,* is a suicide or homicide. Suicide by cop is committing suicide by provoking police to shoot you. Suicide by cop refers to a situation in which police officers will arrive at a scene and the individual purposely disobeys orders from police to lay down his weapon and to surrender. The individual intentionally escalates the potential for the use of force by threatening the police or civilians in the area with a weapon. Officers are then forced to escalate the response.

Suicide by cop is a very lethal method of suicide because the subject knows police officers carry weapons, are trained in the use of guns (and so in all likelihood will kill the target), and will fire in what they perceive to be life-threatening situations. Despite that in the NASH classification it is homicide, it is *not* homicide. (There is something wrong with classifying it as such.)

Geberth (1993) suggested that the two main motives for suicide by cop are that having another kill you lessens the sinfulness of the act and the stigma associated with suicide. (This is especially so in blue cultures.)

Certifications relating to death have four implicit modes or manners of death. The four modes/manners, as we discussed earlier, are natural, accidental, suicide, and homicide; the first letter of each mode makes the acronym NASH. Death certificates categorize accident, suicide, homicide or undetermined; if none apply, the natural category is employed. Of course, the NASH classification of manner of death does not carry the specific mode of such death; for example: "Trauma by bullet (many perforations to the heart) with internal hemorrhage that was caused by a projectile in the chest. The projectile came from the discharge of a firearm's cartridge." This is the immediate cause, not mode. It could be a suicide or homicide, maybe even an accident.

Most deaths are unequivocal; that is, the mode/manner of death is easily certified. Yet there are deaths that are equivocal (i.e., not immediately clear or certain). These are unclear or uncertain deaths; uncertainty can exist between two or more of the modes, such as in some cases of suicide by cop. What then usually occurs is more extensive forensic study of the physical evidence, for example, toxicological reports or DNA testing. But sometimes the designation of the correct manner depends not only on the physical evidence, but on what the deceased had in mind. This is the psychology of the death. Did the person intentionally kill herself? Was she homicidal? Suicidal? The clarification of the mode of death—NASH—centers on the intention of the decedent, what the person "had in mind." The psychological autopsy was devised, as we learned in Chapter 1, to assist in certifying deaths that were ambiguous or undetermined after autopsy, forensic investigation, and so on. It is beyond our intention to discuss suicide by cop in detail (see Lindsay & Lester, 2004, for comprehensive review), but we will discuss some general considerations; the complexities of suicide by cop; concepts of intentionality, lethality and perturbation; a definition of; behavioral, verbal, and contextual clues; and then, the issue of intentionality and understanding in the finality of death.

Historically thus, retrospective investigations were introduced to the field of certification to assist in determining the equivocal cases. The main feature of the psychological investigation is to clarify the equivocal death, namely, what is the correct or accurate mode of death. It is a retrospective investigation of the intention of the deceased (Litman, 1988). Traditionally, there are at least three distinct questions that the psychological autopsy has and can help to answer in suicide by cop:

1. Why did the individual do it?
2. How did the individual die, and when; that is, why at that particular time?
3. What is the most probable mode of death?

Here are first some general considerations to understand suicide and suicide by cop. Marvin Wolfgang (1959) is usually credited with the term "victim-precipitated homicide"; at least Nancy Allen (1980) does so. Wolfgang postulated that such individuals are more like people who die by suicide than like people who die by homicide. They possess characteristics and dynamics most like a person who dies by suicide. One must adopt that point of view to understand them. The difference is the unique means of suicide: by precipitating one's own death.

Wolfgang isolated a number of clues; in all cases the perpetrator was the first to launch an aggressive act, usually with what was perceived to be a lethal weapon. We write *perceived* because not only in Wolfgang's study, but also others, a percentage of cases the *perceived* weapons are not lethal; sometimes a toy gun or BB gun is used. These are typically judged even more to be suicide—the threat was only to self.

The problem in these cases is that the deceased subject precludes direct observation or clinical investigation, but this is also true in all retrospective studies of suicide. We are in *a posteriori* dilemma of study. However, this is common in suicide studies, such as psychological autopsies, since the very beginning of such study, but it can be reliably done.

Wolfgang found that individuals in victim-precipitated homicide cases are willing objects of homicide assaults; that they encourage their own deaths. Although they do not use lethal means/weapons directly on themselves, they are nonetheless, committing suicide. They intentionally (or sometimes subintentionally) have someone else "shoot the gun." Wolfgang presented a number of common characteristics of such individuals: male, lower socioeconomic status, previous arrest record, and psychological and emotional problems.

Incidents in which a suicidal individual engages in conspicuous and threatening behavior in an attempt to get law enforcement to kill him is a phenomenon known as suicide by cop. It is a subtype of victim-precipitated homicide. But is it a homicide? Although "suicide by cop" is a common term, it is more a colloquialism than an accurate description. The victim, or more accurately perpetrator, as the term "victim" should be reserved for those who are truly victims, essentially *forces* the officer to be an unwilling means or instrument in his or her death (Miller, 2006a). It is a suicide. Therefore, there are arguments that suicide by cop may not be the best term. A better term may be "police-forced assisted suicide." However, given the common usage of suicide by cop, we will continue to use this terminology.

It is estimated that about one third of police-involved shootings are suicide by cop (Mohandie, Meloy, & Collins, 2009). The greatest numbers occur in the context of police response to armed robbery. The next most common is response to a domestic violence incident. Miller further noted that a lot of the officers feel manipulated and forced to kill because of the officer's perceived danger in the immediate environment, not necessarily the actual danger. They feared for their safety. Indeed, research suggests that the suicide by cop situations are some of the most stressful that officers face in their careers. The officers are instruments for suicide; otherwise these events are no different from other suicides.

Regarding the complexity of suicide by cop, in the most comprehensive study to date, Kris Mohandie, Reid Meloy, and Peter Collins (2009) examined 707 officer-involved shootings in North America. In this large-scale study, 36% of the officer-involved shootings were found to be suicide by cop. This is well above previous estimates of 10%, suggesting that a large percentage of officer-involved shootings are actually suicides by cop. Mohandie et al. defined suicide by cop as the following, consistent with the definition here:

> "Suicide by cop" is when a subject engages in behavior which poses an apparent risk of serious injury or death, with the intent to precipitate the use of force by law enforcement against the subject. (p. 456)

The three well-known researchers in the forensic field classified each case of the 707 officer-involved shootings, with a high interjudge agreement (with interrater reliability on overall variables being 0.88) for category classified. Thirty-six percent ($n = 256$) were classified as suicide by cop. One-third of these individuals intentionally killed themselves or attempted to kill themselves by having an officer shoot them. The findings confirm the growing incidence of this method of suicide and underscore the significance of suicidal intent among those who become involved in shootings and other force with police officers. Suicide by cop cases were more likely to result in death or injury of the subject than regular officer-involved shooting cases. They are often lethal. Most suicide by cop cases were spontaneous, but had clear verbal and behavioral indications that occurred just prior to and during the event. Suicide by cop individuals had a high likelihood of possessing a weapon (80%, $n = 205$), which were a firearm 60% ($n = 122$) of the time.

Out of 19% (n = 48) who were not armed but feigned or simulated weapon possession, 54% (n = 26) used a replica-type weapon (BB gun, flare gun, etc.). Overall, there was a 97% chance of injury or death to the perpetrator who precipitated those incidents, with a slight majority dying as a result of their encounter with police. Suicide by cop is, thus, a common means of suicide.

Miller (2006a), in his recent review of suicide by cop, noted,

> The crisis episode is commonly precipitated by the rupture of some important relationship in connection with his self-esteem or social support, such as a family or job crisis, that leads to feelings of hopelessness, anger, and despair. Not surprisingly, a desperate reaction is most likely to be provoked where there is a confluence of such crises, such as getting fired and divorced at the same time. (p. 166)

This is true in many suicides. Thus, suicide by cop is no different. It is most like all suicides. It is essentially confusion in certification, largely due to erroneously certifying the death as a homicide. It should, in NASH, even in a medicolegal autopsy, be certified as a *suicide*.

To understand, like all suicides, there is obviously a contextual or situational aspect in suicide by cop. Suicide by cop incidents are complex, multidetermined events. Survivors are generally perplexed, stressed, confused, and even overwhelmed when they are confronted by suicide, and even more so, by suicide by cop. There is such stigma to suicide. A common response by survivors is, thus, that it cannot be a suicide. It is homicide. Like suicide, suicide by cop is, given its complexity, difficult to understand for the layperson, but not the forensic expert or officer. There are at least two reasons why many people do not understand suicide by cop: the very complexity of suicide itself and the fact that suicide is a low frequency event (occurrence) and suicide by cop is even lower, although Mohandie et al. (2009) clearly show that it is much more frequent than often believed.

As we learned, *suicide is a multidimensional event* (Shneidman, 1985; Leenaars, 1996). It is an interplay of individual, relationship, social, cultural, and environmental factors. To understand this better, we need to look at intentionality, lethality, and perturbation in suicide by cop.

Suicide is an intentional act. In suicide, Shneidman (1985) places the emphasis on intentionality, isolating intentioned, subintentioned, and unintentioned death, whether suicide, or as Nancy Allen (1980) showed, homicide.

As we read in Chapter 1, Litman (1984) defined intention as follows:

> The concept, which defines a death as suicide rather than an accident, is intention. For example, we assume that when a man shoots himself in the head with a gun, he intended to die. Therefore the death was a suicide. However, if in fact, he intended to survive, for example, if he thought the gun was not loaded, the death was accidental. (p. 88)

Nancy Allen (1980), in her book, *Homicide*, noted,

> Intentioned homicide, when considered either from the viewpoint of the victim or perpetrator, reflects what direct conscious role was played in effecting the murder. First-degree murder is intended on the part of the perpetrator. The death penalty is considered by courts to be the justifiable intended killing of a person. The "victims" of the death penalty play a role in effecting their own demise and on occasion may murder others, knowing that they are affecting their own death.
>
> Subintentioned homicide occurs when the decedent plays some significant role (even though partial, covert, or unconscious) in hastening his or her own demise. Wolfgang (1958) would refer to this situation as a victim-precipitated homicide. The victim's death is caused partly and sometimes entirely by the role he or she plays in the relationship to his or her killer. The victim, as will be shown in the case histories, uses poor judgment, excessive risk-taking, abuses alcohol or drugs, neglects self, has a self-destructive life style. The individual fosters, facilitates, or hastens his or her death.
>
> The unintentional homicide victim plays no role in effecting his or her own demise. (p. 47)

The characteristics associated with a person predisposed to victim-precipitated homicide are generally defined with suicidal behavior. Lethality helps to define suicide by cop. The higher the lethality in the mind, the more the person intended to die. Parent (1998a) noted that Shneidman (1977) "defines high lethality suicide as the desire to die, a direct and conscious role in bringing about one's own death and that death results primarily due to the decedent's action" (p. 7). In other words, if there is lethal intention to die, it is a suicide (Parent, 1998b). Mohandie et al. (2009) clearly show that intention is very high in suicide by cop cases. Indeed, it is most noteworthy that these well-known forensic experts were able to classify such cases out of 707 officer-involved shooting cases with very high interrater reliability, 88%; it is, thus, not that difficult to do, providing the officer, forensic expert, clinician, and so on, know the clues to look for. There is no question in our mind that incidents of suicide by cop are lethal, not only for the suicidal perpetrator, but also officers, hostages, families, and other people (Mohandie et al. 2009). Thus, we want to know how to predict and control the event. What are the clues?

On March 21, 2009, a "horror," in the words of Acting Chief Howard Jordan, occurred in Oakland California, the worst day in their police history. Lovelle Mixon, a young adult male, killed Officers Mark Dunakin, John Hege, Erv Romans, and Dan Sakal, all respected officers (Oakland Police Shooting: The Mourning After, 2009; Parolee Stood Over Stricken Police Officers and Fired Again, 2009). This was a suicide by cop. The killer, an unemployed ex-felon, was described by his family as "depressed," and determined *never* to return to prison. He was estranged, "lost," and had an extensive criminal record. He was the prime suspect in a rape of a 12-year-old girl. On the traumatic March 21st day, he was stopped for a routine traffic stop, and he is believed to have reacted with other-directed violence. Mixon killed. The situation quickly escalated by him to a suicide by cop, not before he killed more officers, however.

After the first slayings, he ran, with passive supporting cultural/community walls to hide him. Locating in a sister's apartment, police tried to contact Mixon, but there was no response. He killed again! Officers worried about the safety not only for themselves, but also citizens, including the occupants of the apartment. (Was his sister at risk?) Mixon was, we believe, suicidal and chose to end his life by killing officers, and thus, provoking police to shoot him. The officers knew of the deaths and feared for their lives. The Oakland officers were left with no other option but to use deadly force. Mixon had killed, and pointed a weapon, a genuine life-threatening situation. He was shot and killed. This is an extreme case of "homicides among police in suicide by cop."

How does one define and identify suicide by cop? Let us offer a more detailed forensic definition before we look at further clues. Hutson et al. (1998), in one of the first empirical studies on suicide by cop, offer a way of defining such events. They offer a wide array of clues and write,

> Suicidal intent was determined by a written note stating a wish to die, recent verbal communication of a desire to die to friends or family and at times to officers, or exhibiting suicidal characteristics or behavior indicative of suicidal intent (i.e., holding a firearm to one's head). Evidence that suicidal individuals specifically wanted officers to shoot them was determined by the individuals stating outright they wanted officers to shoot them, written or verbal communication to family or friends stating they wanted officers to shoot them, or not dropping their weapon when advised by officers to do so and then aiming their weapon at officers or civilians. (p. 666)

Of course, not all cases include all the clues. They never do. Thus, as in all retrospective investigations, judgments need to be made. Mohandie et al. (2009) suggest that this can be highly reliably done by forensic experts in retrospective investigations and by officers acting in officer-involved shooting cases. Hutson and his team studied all files of officer-involved shooting investigations by the Los Angeles County Sheriff's Department from 1987 to 1997. They found that 11% of officer-involved shootings were suicide by cop, although the incidence is higher in the more current Mohandie et al. study (2009), some 36%. The Los Angeles County Sheriff's Department (LACSD) used the following criteria as a means of identifying suicide by cop incidents:

1. Evidence of suicidal intent
    - Written note stating a wish to die
    - Recent verbal communication of a desire to die to friends or family and at times to officers
    - Suicidal characteristics or behavior indicating suicidal intent (i.e., holding a firearm to one's head)

2. Evidence that suicidal individuals specifically wanted officers to shoot them
   - Outright statements by the precipitators indicating they wanted officers to shoot them
   - Written or verbal communication to family or friends stating they wanted officers to shoot them
3. Refusal to drop their weapon when advised by officers to do so and then aiming their weapon at officers or civilians. Evidence the precipitator possessed a lethal weapon or what appeared to be a lethal weapon.
4. Evidence the precipitator intentionally escalated the encounter and provoked officers to shoot them in self-defense or to protect civilians.

Often times, in a suicide case, not only suicide by cop, we are left asking what behavior clues are present. These may well be life saving for an officer. Lindsay and Lester (2004) in their review of the topic in *Suicide by Cop,* with their insightful subtitle to the topic, *Committing Suicide by Provoking Police to Shoot You* raise the question, "How can police officers decide whether an incident is a suicide-by-cop incident?" Lindsay and Lester provide a list of clues (e.g., behavioral, verbal, contextual; borrowed from Mohandie & Meloy, 2000). The common behavioral clues in suicide by cop, listed by Lindsay and Lester (2004) are as follows (Lindsay & Lester, 2008; Mohandie & Meloy, 2000):

1. demonstrating a weapon
2. pointing the weapon at police
3. clearing an opening in the barricade in order to shoot
4. shooting at police
5. reaching for a weapon with police present
6. attaching the weapon to his/her body
7. counting down to kill hostages or others
8. assaulting or harming hostages
9. forcing a confrontation with police
10. advancing on police when told to stop
11. calling police himself to report a crime in progress
12. continues acts of aggression after being wounded
13. self-mutilation with police present
14. pointing weapon at self
15. refusing to negotiate
16. making no demands to escape
17. making no demands at all
18. getting intoxicated in order to increase his/her courage (p. 18).

The best clue as to suicidal intention, as we learned, is a verbal one. Statements like, "I'm going to commit suicide" are easy to assess; yet about half of suicides do *not* make such statements. Fifty percent do not state, "I'm going to kill myself, "or "Kill me." Twenty percent leave no clue at all. Thus, many suicide by cop cases, but also many suicide cases, are difficult to assess easily. The clues are often not clear and direct; this was the very reason that such investigation began.

Kris Mohandie and Reid Meloy (2000) have also listed a set of verbal clues that indicate that an incident may be suicide by cop. They are

1. demands that the authorities kill him/her
2. setting a deadline for them to kill him/her
3. threatening to kill or harm others
4. wanting to go out in a blaze of glory or indicating that he/she will not be taken alive
5. giving a verbal will
6. telling hostages or others that he/she wants to die
7. looking for a macho way out
8. offering to surrender to the person in charge
9. indicating elaborate plans for his/her own death
10. expressing feelings of depression and hopelessness
11. emphasizing that jail is not an option
12. making Biblical references, especially to the Book of Revelations and resurrection (Lindsay & Lester, 2004, pp. 17–18).

Let us next look at contextual clues. Miller (2006a) writes,

> Immediately prior to a deadly action, the subject may be observed to hyper vigilantly scan the environment or be heard to begin a verbal countdown. Certain actions by the subject may seem to be goading the police into firing at him. He may advance on a police line, after being ordered to stop. He may brandish his weapon in a threatening way, point it at police, clear a threshold in a barricade situation, or actually begin firing; in fact, the latter is the decision point for officers' returning fire in 89% of SBC ('*suicide by cop*') situations studied (Kennedy et al., 1998). Perhaps the most distressing for officers who have killed a SBC subject, he may have been observed reaching for a supposed weapon that turned out to be a toy gun, other harmless object, or just a pantomime intended to manipulate the police into shooting him. (p. 168; italics my insertion)

Like Lindsay and Lester (2004), Miller also noted that there are contextual clues. Among other life problems, he noted that subjects at times had recently sustained a painful traumatic loss or bereavement. Geberth (1993), in fact, speculated that, "Possibly the root of all such occurrences, is the identification the individual has with a parent figure or substitute that has been rejecting and critical" (p. 106). We presented an array of forensic or contextual clues earlier, and will do so throughout this volume.

As discussed earlier, the concept that defines a suicide, including a suicide by cop, is intention. Suicidal intent can be defined as "understanding the physical nature and consequences of the act of self-destruction" (Nolan, 1988, p. 53). There is an understanding of the finality of the self-directed violence. In essence, the retrospective investigation, such as in the psychological autopsy, is nothing less than a thorough study of the intention of the decedent; that is, the person's intention relating to his or her being dead (Shneidman, 1977). The verb "to intend" means to contemplate, to plan, to purpose. The noun, "intention" indicates a psychological exertion for a purpose, to an end (Litman, 1988). Intention is critical; in suicide, there must be intention to die. The person has, in his mind, the intent to be lethal. Litman (1988) stated, "The concept of suicide requires that the self-destructive action has, for at least one of its purposes or goals, the death of the person" (p. 71). Litman (1988) further stated,

> The concept "intentional" signifies to me that the individual in question understood, to some degree, his or her life situation and also understood, to some degree, the nature and quality of the self-destructive action (the proposed action representing to some degree, in the person's mind, killing one's self as a solution to the life situational problem). (p. 72)

He further noted,

> In suicide, a person has it in mind to end a distressing life situation by a self-destructive act, which carries a known predictability for causing death. Death is understood, in the mind of the person, as an end to his or her earthly existence. *When one's own death is being used instrumentally to solve life's problems, we are talking about suicide.* (p. 71)

Thus, the person who intends to die, by Litman's definition, would have to understand the finality of the act. A common question, often asked by people is, How is suicide intent determined? The question is, How can you reach an opinion about what was in the mind of a person who is now dead? Of course, it would be best to ask a person what he or she intended or understood; yet in all cases of suicide, we cannot. This was the very reason that psychological autopsy studies were started. As Nolan (1988) stated,

> Since the suicide victim is dead and unavailable for direct inquiry as to his intention, professionals charged with making such determinations have developed the standard investigatory technique now known as a psychological autopsy. (p. 56)

Litman (1988) makes the further obvious point about intention, even in living people. He stated,

> Unfortunately, absolute certainty about human intentions is seldom achieved even with the living, including our patients, colleagues, and families. We constantly act upon our own evaluations of others' intentions based upon their verbal communications, their behaviors, their previous track records and the social context. (p. 78)

This is what a psychological retrospective study does; it is "an excellent window for viewing and understanding intention" (Litman, 1988, pp. 78–79).

It is a window to what the suicidal person had in mind. And in suicide by cop, what the perpetrator had in mind, as she will kill, to be killed.

As noted earlier, there are exclusions in any argument of intentionality. The most frequent exclusion is the question of "sane, insane." Suicide is an intentional, self-directed act, and many insane people—not all—cannot commit suicide, since that person lacks "the requisite mental capacity to form intent to commit suicide" (Nolan, 1988, p. 52). There are insane people who kill themselves who do not understand the finality of the act. Litman (1988) offers the example of a man who climbed into a lion's area of a zoo under the delusion that he was a biblical prophet with lion-taming powers, but the lion killed him. Often there is no evidence in suicide by cop that the perpetrator was insane, but there is some.

There are further exclusions, such as whether the person's blood-alcohol level is at a significant level that would impair his ability to understand the act. Drug intoxication can be the same. Yet again, they rarely apply. Perpetrators of suicide by cop are intentional suicides, not homicides; although sometimes, they are homicide(s)-suicides. But it should not be confused with suicide among police, although some are suicide by cop in suicide among police.

CONCLUDING REMARKS

It would be accurate to conclude on homicide-suicide something like the following: the offender has a weakened ego, being vulnerable, tends to break down, succeeding to anxiety of rejection and loss. It is a narcissistic injury. The killer becomes overwhelmed by the anticipated loss of love, *the* loved one, or some other ideal. Rejection is central, so is aggression. The perpetrator, whether overcontrolled (like some police cases) or undercontrolled (like most police cases involving domestic violence), rages not only against the rejecting person (or other ideal) but also against the self. He dissociates, a common suicidal state. The walls get higher. All is lost! This is the *Othello Syndrome.*

The ecological model of violence helps us to understand. We believe that suicide and homicide is a stream. We will next explore suicide among police, both classical and current studies, as well as cases of homicide-suicide, including in police.

CHAPTER 3

Police Suicide: Classical Studies

"Suicide in police is at epidemic levels." These were the headlines in the New York media, 1934–1940. Ninety-three New York police officers died by suicide. Anyone who wants to know something about police suicide needs to know about the classical study of the great 1930s suicide epidemic in police. It was the work of one of the world's famous suicidologists, Gregory Zilboorg. It still is a unique but common window to the topic of suicide among police. Yet it does more; Zilboorg's work offers an avenue for the most effective study of police, a psychological autopsy, something still rare in the psychological investigation of police suicide.

Shneidman helped to create at least two major endeavors in suicidology: the psychological autopsy, which is intended to clarify the psychological nature of a death and postvention, pertaining to the care of the bereaved.

The concept of investigating deaths, which are uncertain as to mode of death—natural, accident, suicide, or homicide—is at least as old as the work of John Graunt of London in the 17th century. The recent history of this procedure focuses around the Los Angeles Suicide Prevention Center (LASPC). In the 1950s, the Chief Coroner and Medical Examiner of Los Angeles County, Theodore Curphey, asked the leaders at the LASPC—Edwin Shneidman, Norm Farberow, and Robert Litman—to assist him with coroners' cases that were ambiguous as to the mode of death, usually between accident and suicide, but sometimes homicide. These were cases dependent upon the decedent's *intention*. The Center's three leaders were designated as deputy coroners and went to the scenes of death, where they gently interviewed a number of key survivors. They then reported back to Dr. Curphey in a setting that was strictly nonpartisan, that is, no one had a brief for one mode of death of another (e.g., homicide or suicide). This chapter presents detailed psychological autopsies by Gregory Zilboorg and his team, of the 1930s epidemic of police suicide, provides an outline for the retrospective psychological investigative procedure, presents the findings (or evidence), and makes suggestions for the prevention of such deaths. There is a rich trove of suggestions, few ever followed since.

After a suicide has been committed, the tragedy is not over. Shneidman coined the word "postvention" to refer to those activities that can assuage the grief and

http://dx.doi.org/10.2190/SHSC3

mollify the mourning processes of the survivor-victims. The latter part of the chapter, on the care of the bereaved, sets forth the findings of the aftershocks (the sting) in the survivors of the New York police suicides, some 50 years later, by Jack Kamerman. The pain continues; largely because more needed to be done. Dissembling and masking occurred. There is, of course, enormous *stigma* to have an emotional disturbance (psychopathology) and to kill oneself, especially among police. This stigma was/is/will be suicidogenic. The next chapter, on current studies of suicide among police, shows this fact!

* * * * * *

INTRODUCTION

"Suicide in police is at epidemic levels." These were the headlines in the New York media, 1934–1940. Ninety-three New York policemen committed suicide (Friedman, 1967a). Anyone who wants to know something about police suicide needs to know about this classical study. It is a window to the topic. It offers a unique opportunity to understand suicide in a select group of people "who would be attracted to the career of making their livelihood through police work" (p. 414).

Before we summarize, Friedman stated that one must know a few historical facts. He writes,

> 1. The psychological atmosphere that existed in New York in the 1920s, especially during the years 1925–1927, was a period of Tammany control. It was a time of protection by a political boss, the so-called "rabbi," who not only got a man placed on the police force, but acted as the source through which the patrolman once on the force obtained special assignments and became part of a system of accepting and dispensing graft and gratuities. One obvious implication of this historical fact is that the standards of competence or stability were obviously not always the criteria for selection to a police department.
> 2. The second relevant historical fact concerns the impact of the changes in the psychological atmosphere within the New York Police Department that followed the election (in 1933) of Fiorello La Guardia as mayor. These changes affected particularly the status of the police officer who was overly aggressive, alcoholic, or profligate—many of whom had been tolerated (or even unconsciously encouraged) in the police department during the pre-La Guardia era. (pp. 415–416)

The suicide rate among policemen had, indeed, reached alarming levels and triggered public interest. Inspector Neidig received specialized attention publicly and among the service itself. Neidig, a 52-year-old well-respected officer, had been 4 years in command of a most important division. He was a public figure. He shot and killed himself with his service revolver after a series of painful personal and departmental events. The *New York Post* reported on his death and especially called for independent investigation. "Why did the suicide occur?" the editor asked.

INVESTIGATIONS: A PSYCHOLOGICAL AUTOPSY

Mayor La Guardia ordered a special investigation, what we now call "psychological autopsies." The suicidologist that he called on was Gregory Zilboorg, one of the top 10 classical suicidological theorists, and his team (the Committee for the Study of Suicide). A public report was released; among other matters, it presented the findings of Inspector Neidig's psychological autopsy. One of Zilboorg's first acts of postvention was, in fact, to publish a letter to the *New York Post*, to teach people what suicide is, including the specific case of Neidig. He wrote,

> Generalizations on reasons for suicide prove as a rule as inadequate as generalizations for such predilections as liking strawberries. Each individual case presents its own story and its own reasons. While the story of Inspector Neidig is not fully known, it appears more than significant that only recently his brother and mother were carried away by a serious illness. People symbolically joining their dead by means of suicide are more frequent than one would be inclined to suspect. Seemingly unmotivated suicides on the anniversaries of relatives' deaths or on some other occasions which revive the memory of a departed close relative are not infrequent. One single motivation almost never leads to a suicidal act. Usually it is a combination of motivations which we, in our technical language, call constellations of motives. The fact that of recent years there have been a number of suicides among policemen is undoubtedly of great sociological importance; also, the fact that this "suicidal period" appears to roughly coincide with the anti-racketeering crusade is suggestive. The law and crime have marginal connections. The fringes of both margins intermingle. The law officer, even the most serene and conscientious, carries within him a complicated psychological structure; while defending the integrity of society and the safety of its citizens, he, like a soldier, must do it through extreme mobilization of his inner powers of aggression which he always keeps available to work. In time he gets disciplined or otherwise faces a situation in which he must submit instead of pushing others into submission; his aggression becomes dammed up and turns upon the individual himself. That is the reason why, perhaps, there are more suicides during peace time than during wars and revolutions, for in peace time the individual has much fewer direct outlets for his inner aggressions. That is why, incidentally, such a country as Germany has always showed a greater number of suicides than any other nation in the world and a smaller number of murders in proportion; for the Germans have been preeminently living in a psychological state of passive submission. On the other hand, when the would-be suicide succeeds in finding an outlet for his aggression he presents to us a picture of running a Hitlerian amok. It is not therefore impossible that Inspector Neidig, like many of his colleagues, fell victim to this internalized aggression; that is, he shot himself when he couldn't shoot his boss. (pp. 419–420)

Zilboorg's insights are worth remembering as we attempt to understand the occurrences in front of us today.

Psychological autopsies were completed; the following is a sampling of what Zilboorg learned about the 93 suicidal policemen:

- 75% of the group were married
- Although all ranks were represented (sergeant, lieutenant, captain, inspector, and deputy inspector), 64% were patrolmen
- 22% had a history of alcoholism
- 29% had a history of a mental health diagnosis (20 had a neurosis, 3 had psychosis, 2 had a personality disorder)
- 5% were homicide-suicides
- 90% used their service gun
- The psychological and social factors of being a "cop" were determined to be significant.

There are a number of other relevant ecological factors before the La Guardia era. The gun was deemed central, and the belief/attitude in the New York force was "To deprive a man of a gun was unusual unless he was truly violent or disgraceful dismissal." There was no gun control, a lethal situation. Domestic violence, a common factor, was prevalent, but also was ignored; wives' complaints to the department were hidden. Suicidal clues, such as verbal statements, "If I got broken, I'd take to the gas pipe (suicide)," were ignored. There was no prevention. Psychological and social maladjustments were tolerated. There was no mental health service or support, and if there was, it enabled the suicidal atmosphere. The New York force was running amok.

After La Guardia, as noted, the "amok" atmosphere changed. Order was implemented; yet many were upset, perturbed, and agitated. One officer stated, "Now the public can and does hate cops—and don't cops know it."

Domestic violence was not tolerated. Wives could complain and action was taken. This resulted in not only an increase in frustration, aggression, and hostility, but also an increase in homicide-suicides. There was great fear that one could lose one's gun, one's revolver. And, in one case, after a mistress was publicly revealed, Friedman (1967) wrote, "One threatened in this way shot and killed his wife and himself" (p. 426). Alcoholism also increased. Violence, both inwardly and outwardly directed, also increased.

Another change that came about was in relation to the service revolver. Before, reckless and inappropriate use of the gun was tolerated, now gun control was instituted. Friedman writes,

> Now suspicion of dangerous careless behavior could mean deprivation of the gun. As one who was deprived of a gun remarked, "I felt so ashamed, so helpless. I was not a cop any more." The gun is more than an implement of the policeman's trade; it is a symbol of his power. Guns may be taken away during periods of suspension or even of censure. To many this deprivation was the greatest possible disgrace. (p. 427)

Zilboorg, based on his psychological autopsies, concluded the following:

> In summary, all the deprivations listed above, frustrations, and ego-deflationary situations, combined with the more exacting demands for honest police work, disturbed the depth of the personality of the insecure, unstable, and immature policeman, who was so thoroughly affected that it made his whole living plan one of evident maladjustment. These maladjustments varied in their manifestations according to the original type of personality in its self-indulging days before the change in regime. The "breakdowns" were predominantly psychotic among the passive and insecure but "good cops" and were explosively delinquent and, in some instances, murderous among the aggressive, immature personalities with their bases of disturbed marital life, serious alcoholism, and complete dependence for primary gratification on an organization that had allowed them to exploit aggressive personality patterns.
>
> One must not overlook the fact, however, that it was the original unstable, insecure, and immature core of the policeman's personality that was at fault and not the new regime and its exactions. To repeat, the disappearance of the loose police organization and its involved political affiliations that had previously provided outlets that enabled this type of individual to function and the substitution of a stringent system forced upon him impotence and destruction of his whole living program. Should he seek meaning and fulfillment in his family and through the usual means of everyday life and relationships, he failed again, because these sources had never been utilized and the relationships had never been built on the basis of a sound, mature personality. In the vernacular, he had placed all his eggs in one basket (the Police Department and gratification as a policeman), and the bottom fell out.
>
> With the change, the hostile and aggressive policeman who formerly functioned with social license suddenly began to feel like a frustrated child. No one would support him, and everyone was against him or was unsympathetic. Some "took it out" on themselves by extreme alcoholism and illness; others, by aggressive and murderous acts—all eventually leading to so much pent-up murderous hostility as to eventuate in suicide. The latter type was vividly illustrated in the case of the policeman who waited for hours to kill the sergeant he hated. When the sergeant failed to appear, the policeman killed himself. (Friedman, 1967a, pp. 427–428)

OVERVIEW OF PSYCHOLOGICAL PROBLEMS

The findings of the psychological autopsies were most revealing about the psychological facts; thus, we again quote verbatim in detail:

> A detailing of the lives of these ninety-three policemen, especially before their acceptance by the Police Department, may furnish significant clues of the act of suicide. A surprisingly large number—63 of the 93 (67 percent) manifested some behavior trait that indicated mental imbalance. The majority of this group were obviously psychotic, of either the depressive or paranoic type. Two-thirds of the cases included in the group of psychotic,

> prepsychotic, or seriously neurotic types were essentially passive individuals who were frequently of the quiet, reliable, and, in many cases, inadequate or inconsequential personalities whose suicide on superficial examination seemed to have no obvious cause. However, the majority of them during most of their lives had been good examples of "home men," "good cops," and superficially adjusted personalities. They had generally been well-liked, most often just "one of the gang"; most of them had not been extreme alcoholics, and they had exemplified a superficially satisfactory marital adjustment. In periods ranging from a few months to a few years before their suicides, a disintegration of personality developed. Their fellow policemen recognized in only a few instances that their friend was under some strain or stress. Those who became extremely alcoholic, the "rummies," were protected by their fellow workers because of their previously good reputations. Camaraderie that is usually restrained came to the fore after the breakdown, and the good cop or good fellow was helped on all sides. Superior officers, police surgeons, and fellow policemen did not want to see him lose his job. Consequently, his benefactors, because of both their desire to help and their ignorance of the nature of his severe mental illness, nursed him along instead of encouraging him to go on the sick list. This procedure was very evident. It was usually not until their mental illness had become very severe that they were treated as "queer" or "sick."
>
> Others of this group, who had for years been the good cops, suddenly developed irritable, suspicious, or despondent behavior. An examination of their home life betrayed a psychopathy which must have been quiescent and of long standing and which had burst forth in a psychosis just before the suicide.
>
> One-third of this mentally unstable and psychotic group were of an overtly aggressive, impulsive, and reckless nature. There was a high percentage of alcoholics among them. Those in the passive group had been predominantly functioning policemen who had had some degree of adjustment prior to their mental breakdown and eventual suicide, whereas in the aggressive group the life plan had been one of maladjustment in relation to work, family, and self.
>
> The incidence of alcoholics was higher and the extent of indulgence in alcohol was greater in the aggressive group. Among them, 70 percent were severe alcoholics whereas only 36 percent of the passive group were.
>
> Whereas 64 percent of the aggressive group were most frequently involved in marital discord, only 26 percent of the passive group failed to make an acceptable marital adjustment. Further, of the aggressive group only one could have been called a good cop with regard to character and efficiency as a policeman, whereas 57, or 70 percent, of the passive group had been respected as good cops by their commanding officers.

The aggressive group was of special interest; we continue with the quote:

> Two-fifths of the total group coming within this aggressive, assertive personality type showed a lower incidence of psychotic or prepsychotic trend than did the passive group. However, during their life activity prior to the suicide, they did manifest a greater personality disorganization. Persistent

and severe alcoholism, greater marital discord, loose sexual living, and precarious security as a policeman were so vividly the pattern that a frequently heard statement from or about these men was "the digging of their own graves." Often they themselves felt that this grave-digging process was inflicting harm on their friends or family, and the suicide itself was reacted to by these relatives with an awareness that the suicide was the final *coup de grâce* of aggression. Many widows commented, "Why did he do this to me?" "How could he leave me this way?" etc. Just over half this group showed in their suicide anger or aggression toward their wives, and often in their suicide notes expressed unrestrained hostility toward them. Some even forbade their wives to attend the funeral. A large number of these actually committed the act after a violent argument with, or following a series of frustrations by, their spouse. A number were threatened by the wife with exposure in police headquarters of their extramarital sexual behavior, wife-beating, excessive drinking, and, in a few instances, irregular police behavior. The frequency of murder threats in this group was high. Examples were:

One young policeman, alcoholic, with a bad record on the force, had been carrying on extramarital sexual relations. He impregnated a girl and married her in a pompous church ceremony, set up another home, and tried to keep the secret from both wives while living with each. The first wife discovered the bigamy but was restrained from revealing it for fear her husband would shoot her as he had often threatened. Her mother, however, betrayed him. He pulled his gun and wanted to shoot both the woman and her mother. Then, telling his wife that his suicide was inevitable, he was further angered by her taunting refusal to believe that he would do it. He shot himself then and there.

Another patrolman, when threatened by his wife with exposure of his various mistress relationships, shot and killed her and then himself. He was known in his district as "king of the beat;" in the station house his fellow patrolmen were afraid of his temper but flattered him by calling him "stud horse."

One patrolman, on the force for ten years, married twice, frequently up for disciplinary charges, often intoxicated while on and off duty, beat and abused his wife and was always accusing her of infidelity. He himself was suspected of considerable extramarital sexual activity. On at least one occasion, in a fit of temper, he shot at a fellow patrolman. His suicide occurred after he shot and killed a policeman who refused to drink with him.

Other cases of this nature can be enumerated. At least half (eighteen) and probably more of the aggressive group were known to have recklessly fired their guns or threatened frequently to fire and kill. At least five had murdered someone just before their suicide.

This picture of maladjustment had been evident long before they joined the Department: Vocational status had been one of considerable insecurity; jobs had been in the unskilled and semiskilled fields and had been held for only a short time; economic status had been low; alcoholism was not infrequent. In a number of cases minor delinquencies were evident, whereas in a few cases actual arrests for assaultive behavior were on record. (pp. 429–432)

The case studies reveal the idographic, the individual. There were cases of planned or committed homicide-suicide in the group. We here offer a few examples of the police suicides; they allow us to understand the suicidal police officer better. We here present some examples verbatim of the Friedman text:

> We have the case of another patrolman, 37 years of age, married twice, and on the force for seven years. His first marriage was one of much quarrelling, with flaunting infidelity on the part of both. There is, further, an allusion in his record to promiscuous sexual behavior before this first marriage and to an illegitimate child whose support he had to guarantee before he could get on the force.
>
> His first marriage was of a nature suggesting coercion on the wife's part, with resultant discord. His fellow patrolmen frequently claimed that his wife had sexual relations with other patrolmen in her husband's precinct. Divorce followed after much difficulty.
>
> His seven years on the police force was such as to elicit from some men in his station house the remark, "He was no loss to the Department." In his record he is reported to have shot himself while cleaning his gun. From some informed sources this incident appears to have been the result of a quarrel with his wife, concerning which he angrily remarked, "I almost shot her at the time."
>
> Seven months after his divorce and about eighteen months before his suicide, he remarried. His friends claim that he was again disappointed and unhappy in marriage, "since his wife was lavish and she expected him to support her folks."
>
> In his precinct he was surly, irritable, and disliked. He often remarked that everyone was against him. Toward a certain sergeant he was especially angry. He felt hounded by him and not infrequently fearful of being brought up on charges of either drinking or negligent police duty.
>
> On the day of the suicide he felt especially plagued by the sergeant, and after finishing his tour he went to a barroom where he waited for the sergeant to appear. To some people in the saloon he said that he was going to kill the officer as soon as he saw him. For some time he waited impatiently, frequently going to the street to look for him. After a long while he returned to his barroom table and wrote the following note, which he addressed to the same sergeant:
>
> "Sergeant:
>
> "Goodbye you old prick and when I mean prick you are a prick. Hope you fall with the rest of us, you yellow bastard.
>
> May the [number of the precinct] get along without you."
>
> Although the note implies that some disclosure about the sergeant's affairs might be made, there has been no such disclosure. However, the sergeant later seemed to have been paranoid. (pp. 438–439)

On a note, obviously homicide-suicide among police was already a fact.

A case of another officer:

> An example is the case of a patrolman, forty-five years of age, who had an excellent record for twenty-two years on the force, was married, had two children, and lived close to a large clannish family. He was the eighth of nine children born of a stern father and capable mother who dominated the whole household. His father died of cancer when the patrolman was twenty-two. He was his mother's favorite. She died of a kidney ailment when he was twenty-seven. As a child and an adult he lived an active, happy life, although somewhat dominated more by the girls of the family than the other boys. He stopped school at sixteen to enter the family trade of stonecutting. He entered the Police Department only after being urged by relatives on the force and passed the police examination despite himself. He was proud of being a policeman and was well-known for his fastidiousness and regard to work, appearance, and family life. Always overprotective of his two daughters, who "adored" him, he blocked their too-intimate contact with boys, saying "There isn't anything a boy can give you that I can't." His married life was said to be "very happy."
>
> After an appendectomy, eight years before his suicide, he developed what he and others called "writer's cramp." He was very sensitive about this and always borrowed others' pens and pencils, with the thought that he could control his writing better with them. Some months before the suicide he angrily tossed a pen to the floor, saying, "Damn it, my writing is like a kid's." Between his thirty-eighth and forty-fifth year, four of his siblings died, the last death, nine months before his suicide, being that of his favorite sister.
>
> Three months later "he just seemed to mope around the house." He suffered from constipation and feared cancer. His medical record had a notation of a gastric neurosis for which he received the usual medical treatment. The last six months of his life he worked at his job but was said "to be in a fog." The night before his death, while trying to write a note, he very angrily threw his pencil away again, saying that his was child's writing. The next morning, after shaving and inquiring about his daughter who had just started her first job, he shot and killed himself.
>
> This case is presented at greater length because it is a good example of the life and work of so many of the group who were spoken of as reliable, passive, and good policemen.

And in another case:

> There was one patrolman, thirty-seven, single, on the force for nine years, who had not only a good police record but a reputation among his fellow workers for being a good friend and worthwhile person.
>
> He shot himself after writing a note leaving his considerable savings to his sister and close male friend. In the note he said that he suffered from such severe headaches that he could not go on, and further, that "before I do something that may hurt someone else, this is the best way out."
>
> His father had been committed to an insane asylum repeatedly after sexually attacking his own daughter (the patrolman's twin sister) when she was about twelve years of age. A few days before the patrolman's suicide, he visited his father in the institution. Upon his return home he was said to

> have been exceptionally depressed at finding his father so insane as to be unable to recognize him.
>
> The headaches that the patrolman suffered so severely were unknown to his police surgeon, and the medical record shows no awareness of the man's physical or mental condition.
>
> His suicide was one that evoked from all who knew him the statement, "We would never believe it. . . . He had everything. . . . There was no reason for his doing it. (pp. 439–441)

Dissembling and masking were common. Even when there was identified risk, nothing was done. Family and fellow officers hesitated to do anything, even covering up domestic violence. Yet this proved to be lethal. Friedman (1967a) wrote,

> In a few cases in which the patrolman was thought to be acting queerly, his family and friends hesitated to have him see the psychiatrist, or "nut doctor," as the average policeman called him. To most police families and men on the force, referral to the psychiatrist or neurologist meant almost certain discharge from the Department. Not only was there a reluctance to refer a man to what was felt to be his "doom," but in most instances his breakdown was never recognized. (pp. 441–442)

On masking with and by others, Friedman wrote:

> This is one of the few instances on record of the mental disturbances being so aggravated as to bring the patrolman to a psychiatrist. But, as is evident even in this instance, the authorities were always too reluctant to recognize the seriousness of the man's illness, because it could mean causing him to lose his job. Although policemen are quite commonly suspicious of each other and are careful to keep their private affairs secret, they become overprotective when a fellow worker is in difficulty. In fact, in some instances, even serious misdemeanors are covered up, and this overprotective relationship holds for the attitude of superior officers toward the men in the ranks as well as for the attitude of the patrolmen toward one another. (p. 443)

Of course, there was enormous stigma to have a mental disorder, no different from today. On this, Friedman wrote,

> One manner of handling the mentally or physically ill patrolman was to take him away from regular duty. This most frequently meant placing him on the duty called "raided premises," which usually consisted of guarding raided houses or hotels used by prostitutes. The purpose appeared to be that of keeping prostitutes from again inhabiting the place. The patrolman sat quietly by himself in one spot for a full eight-hour shift. In other instances, the recipient of light duty was given a simple errand or clerical job. In the case of both assignments, the average policeman felt much contempt for the job and condescending sympathy for those assigned to it. Some of our cases avoided and feared these assignments, saying, "I'll be damned if I'll cut paper dolls all day." As one said, "It's the next step to the nut house." One

> patrolman who felt that he was being "discriminated" against refused an inside assignment with the words, "That's no job for a man." In his disturbed behavior he thought people were claiming that he was "not a man." (p. 443)

This is suicidogenic for officers! This continues.

This does not mean that on occasion, an officer with a mental disorder was not spotted; yet, proper psychological action or prevention, was not taken. Rather, Friedman observed,

> The incidence of probable psychotic breakdown of all the cases is higher in this good-cop group. They were occasionally spotted by the police surgeon who too often used the diagnoses of gastric neurosis, neurosis, anxiety neurosis, and neurasthenia and too frequently impatiently urged the patrolman back to duty. Even when the surgeons were more sympathetic, no significant psychiatric treatment was given in any except two cases which were sent to psychiatric sanatoriums.
>
> The incipient mental breakdown or suicidal impulses in the good-cop group were not easy for either the police surgeon or fellow patrolmen to detect. However, most of those close to the man knew that something was wrong with him. (p. 439)

Could the dissembling have been better detected? And even if the health professional or supervisor knew, could something more have been done? Zilboorg, in fact, made some implemented life-saving recommendations. The 1940 questions are still in front of us today. Could better prevention have been utilized? What are the best ways to intervene with a suicidal police officer? A homicidal-suicidal police officer? Could we, aspiring to rescue, have prevented the officer's suicide? The questions are the same as asked by Gregory Zilboorg many years ago.

SURVIVING THE GREAT SUICIDE EPIDEMIC IN POLICE

The survivors—how did they adjust to one of the worst possible traumas? On this question, we are fortunate, due to the psychological autopsies, to be able to provide some answers, not only immediately, but also many years later (Kamerman, 1993). Jack Kamerman has, in fact, interviewed the survivors of the New York police suicides decades later. First, however, a few comments on survivorship in general.

The pain of the suicide becomes the pain of the survivor. Anguish, guilt, anger, sadness, shame, and anxiety are a sample of the pains. Arnold Toynbee (1968) makes the point that death is a two party event. He writes,

> The two-sidedness of death is a fundamental feature of death—not only of the premature death of the spirit, but also of death at any age and in any form. There are always two parties to a death; the person who dies and the survivors who are bereaved.

> The sting of death is less sharp for the person who dies than it is for the bereaved survivor.
>
> This, as I see it, is the capital fact about the relation between living and dying. There are two parties to the suffering that death inflicts; and in the apportionment of this suffering, the survivor takes the brunt. (pp. 327–332)

Toynbee here resonates Saint Paul's question, "O death, where is thy sting?" As we see it, the brunt is even more for the survivors of suicide. This suffering is even greater. The inflicting is more intentional. There are deep feelings of rejection, often perceived as the ultimate one (van der Wal, 1989–90). There is frequently a belief that the sting was malicious (Clark & Goldney, 1995). Survivors ask, "Did she want me to hurt so?"

Suicide is a dyadic event. It is a relationship. Shneidman (1972) noted,

> I believe that the person who commits suicide puts his psychological skeletons in the survivor's emotional closet—he sentences the survivor—to deal with many negative feelings and, more, to become obsessed with thoughts regarding his own actual or possible role in having precipitated the suicidal act or having failed to abort it. It can be a heavy load. (p. 10)

The load is indeed a heavy burden; the skeletons live. The "extent of the problem" has only been recognized in the last 10 to 15 years. There has, in fact, been a rapidly growing effort by many—professionals, psychologists, social workers, psychiatrists, nurses, and the lay public—to understand the skeletons, the problem. Yet there are taboos, walls, and these were even more so in the 1940s.

Kamerman has been studying the families of those New York police officers, "the survivors who have lived with the legacies of their deaths." In a unique study, the families have been followed for over 60 years now. The main conclusion: The suicides of the police officers "have affected the lives of wives, sons, and daughters, grandchildren and great-grandchildren." There is such pain. Indeed, for some, "the suicide became the central organizing event in their lives." Yet for others, they learned to survive, requiring painful adjustment, but for some, just living their lives. However, for all there was a family *illegacy*. How will an officer's homicide-suicide affect the lives of family, friends, fellow officers, and the public?

Maybe the insights gained from the survivors of the New York police officers can guide us. Kamerman offers some unique insights. He writes,

> In all cases of children interviewed so far, they maintained, from their own memories or on the basis of what they had been told . . . that their fathers loved them very much, treated them well, and were in general model parents.
>
> Just as with the romanticization of their marriages, widows tended to rework over time the circumstances leading up to their husbands' suicides. Of course, if professionals sometimes puzzle over the causes of a suicide, widows also might have trouble understanding it. Every widow I spoke to had a theory as to why her husband had killed himself. In only one of my

interviews with widows did the widow see herself involved in the causative chain, and then not really in a way that would likely be construed as blameworthy.

> I never really found out the true story. I never really found out the truth because, I don't know what it was, there seemed to be such a blockage in my head, and I didn't want to . . . the things I was thinking of, I didn't want to hear, anyhow. And it was never brought up. . . . The only thing I was afraid of was, maybe he had a drink, going in [to work]. And maybe they smelled liquor on him. And then he was so afraid of me hearing, or that I'd be annoyed about it or something, and this is what he'd done. I don't *know*. That's only *my thoughts*. I don't know. Other than that I don't know. [Interview with widow, November 1989]

In other cases, problems related to the job or to things going on in the husband's psyche constituted their explanations of their husbands' suicides.

> Well, it was a shock, that is all. And I mean, nothing to explain it, you know. The only thing—this is a very, very personal thing—the only thing I can think of is be became . . . incompetent? Incontinent? No— the sex business . . . What is the word? [Interviewer: Impotent.] Impotent, yet, isn't that awful—Yes. That's the only thing. And that was only in the last couple of weeks before he died. Now, whether that affected him or not, I don't know. He didn't go to a doctor. He went to the . . . the . . . oh, what is the big thing the police give at Christmas time? When they go . . . the Holy Name Society. He went to that, and he was dead on the twentieth [of December]. [Interview with widow. 21 November 1989]

According to the records from the 1940 study, in the first case there had been no drinking, but the officer had had a disciplinary charge brought against him for being off his post. In the second case, the officer had been brought up on a disciplinary charge that had been resolved the day before his suicide with an apology to the offended citizen. In the 1940 interview, his widow had mentioned the suspension of sexual activities shortly before the suicide, but didn't see it as related to the suicide. Instead she pointed to the disciplinary hearing and the fact that he had become nervous and had experienced a buzzing in his head, which had led to an appointment with a police physician, as the only things that might have had a connection with his suicide. It is difficult to decide from the interviews done so far the extent to which the suicide has become part of family lore passed down from generation to generation (pp. 353–354).

CONCLUDING REMARK

What will be the police suicide's lore?

CHAPTER 4

Police Suicide: Current Studies

What is the current lore about police suicide? The classical studies of New York continue to impact the current ones. Many of the questions raised continue. Is there a suicide epidemic in police? What are the causes? Can we study the events? How? Psychological autopsies? There are many questions. In this chapter, we answer some that confront us today and tomorrow.

Fact: Suicide among police occurs. Yet is it at epidemic levels? There are answers. And fact: Homicide-suicide in police occurs. And it can be shown that homicide-suicide is well above the statistical probability. Homicide-suicide among police is at epidemic levels. Is emotional disturbance relevant? Is depression? Is alcoholism? Is domestic violence relevant? Are interpersonal problems relevant? Was there loss and rejection? Was there work-related loss, a loss of the gun, for example? Are guns frequently used? There are many more facts than in the 1930s. Yet there is one critical problem: the lack of evidence continues. We lack *evidence*.

This chapter presents the work of Bruce Danto (working on suicide in the Detroit Police Service), Robert Loo (studying suicide in Canada's Royal Canadian Mounted Police [RCMP]), John Violanti (presenting the largest informative array of police studies; we owe him much in the field; he is a grandfather of forensic suicidology in police), and Peter Marzuk (presenting probably the best study today, once more among New York police). The verdict on the question, *Is it an epidemic?:* to the best of our current understanding, and despite not knowing everything (a constant in forensic investigation anyway), an answer is provided. Yet many questions remain to be answered. Like many others, including ours, Violanti's solution: Allow for intensive study of police suicide.

The study of suicide among police has, however, increasingly not been allowed. Some things remain the same since the New York epidemic of 1934–1940. Why?

Although Gregory Zilboorg asked the question, it was probably Bruce Danto, 30 years ago, who most forcefully asked: "Is it significant that so little personal information was available?" Was there masking? This is called *dissembling*, so suicidogenic in police, but pervasive. Psychological autopsies are not allowed. There are blue barriers, what Danto called "blue walls." Yet the walls affect not only study but also getting help. Danto found a lack of psychological services for

http://dx.doi.org/10.2190/SHSC4

at-risk officers. Does this continue today? In fact, in a rare study, Ann-Marie Berg, and her team from Norway, showed the evidence about help-seeking in police. The suicidal officer does not go for help! Is this due to the blue culture, the stigma? Zilboorg, Danto, and other forensic experts say, *yes*. We believe so. *Therefore*: Nothing is going to get done until the blue walls come down.

We believe: We can understand suicide among police better. And, if we do, we can understand homicide-suicide in police better. They can be predicted and prevented, only if police have a will to do so.

* * * * * *

INTRODUCTION

The classical studies of New York continue to impact the current studies. Many of the questions raised continue. There are, of course, more recent tragedies. It is estimated, by National Police Suicide Foundation (NPSF), that about 400 police officers die by suicide in the United States every year (we do not know in Canada.) That would be 2 to 3 times the number killed in line of duty. However, the NSPF, an organization for the prevention of police suicide in the United States, obtains its data voluntarily from newspapers and the like. There is no national systematic mortality data registry. We predict, based on the research, that the rates are higher, much higher. On October 2, 2008, for example, a family man and respected New York police officer, Michael Pigott, on his 46th birthday, died by suicide. Lt. Pigott was involved in a September 24th case in which police fired a Taser gun at Iman Morales, an emotionally disturbed man. Lt. Pigott had ordered the use of the Taser. Subsequent to Morales' death, Lt. Pigott was being investigated for violation of department guidelines, stripped of his badge and gun and placed on modified duties. Fearing that his career would never be the same, Lt. Pigott publicly apologized. He was reported to be "torn up" by the occurrence, and on October 2, 2008, took a service pistol from another officer's locker and shot himself at the station. He left a suicide note stating, "It was all my fault," adding that "he didn't want his kids to see him cuffed and jailed." A fellow officer stated, "When they pulled the carpet out from under him, it destroyed his whole world." Thus, Pigott's family, fellow officers, and we are left to ask, Is there a suicide epidemic in police? What are the causes? Can we study the events? How? There are many questions that confront us today.

One of the most obvious facts is that yes, there are suicides in police. Yet is it at epidemic levels? An epidemic according to the OED is: "Of a disease: normally absent or infrequent in a population but liable to outbreaks of greatly increased frequency and severity." It is widespread or prevalent. Further, there are homicide-suicides in police. At least, it can be shown that this is well above the standard population. Is domestic violence relevant? Yes. Are guns frequently used? Yes. There are many more insights than those gained in the 1940s. However, there is one continuing critical problem: the lack of data continues. We lack evidence.

INVESTIGATIONS OF POLICE SUICIDE

For an early example, Bruce Danto (1978), a psychiatrist and an officer, studied the suicides in police in Detroit, Michigan. Like in New York, there had been a rash of suicides in the police force in Detroit. Twelve officers, all male, committed suicide from February 1968 to January 1976. They were from all ranks. Danto was called on to study the deaths; yet he quickly noted that there was a paucity of data. He asked if data were hidden. Was there masking? He wrote, "Is it significant that so little personal information was available?" (p. 34). He noted that insights would be limited and called for psychological autopsies, but it "was not possible to perform a psychological autopsy on the deceased officers." This is a pity. Unfortunately this continues to be the case, as we will learn. There are blue barriers.

In his study, Danto noted that his findings were similar to the New York police officers in many ways. Marital or relationship problems were figural; these were precipitating events, in fact. Many had a history of alcoholism. Firearms were the preferred method. Relationship problems/disharmony before the death was common. Work stresses were also implicated. For an officer, Danto concluded that to some extent "problems may be consistent to his work because his hours are erratic, constantly subject to change, and the officer is subjected to danger which is beyond the reach of most civilian minds" (p. 36). Be that as it may, the vast majority of the suicides were committed "in response to important personal problems." Similar to New York, there was sound evidence of emotional disturbances ("neurosis"), especially "anxiety and depressive symptoms." A long history of personality problems was evident and associated with maladjustment. Danto did observe differences. He did not find such a high presentation of aggression. He also did not believe, as suggested by Zilboorg in his reports, that aggressive people chose the profession of a police officer. Yet the incident of homicide-suicide was very high. One third of the suicides were homicides-suicides. That is epidemic! He writes,

> Murder followed by suicide was the pattern in 4 of the cases, but in one case, the suicide occurred two months later. In 2 of those cases, the murder victim was a wife, in another the victim was an ex-husband of his wife, and in the last case the victim was a bar owner with whom the officer had argued in a bar. It would be possible to state that guilt feelings and fear of punishment were involved in these 4 cases; this need not be the case. In one murder-suicide there had been considerable guilt feeling expressed by the officer about killing two suspects in the line of duty. (p. 35)

Is that true? Do homicide-suicides occur more frequently in police officers than the general population? If so, this has huge implications for what we do for suicidal officers. Is domestic violence relevant? And if not, are disturbing or troubling relations relevant? What does the research say?

One of the most disturbing findings by Danto was again the lack of services for at-risk officers. Is this related to what are called blue walls (barriers) to help-seeking? Danto, however, also noted that officers often report that there are "locked doors" by professionals. He wrote,

> In the eyes of many officers with whom I talked, the psychiatrist talks down to the officer. His lack of sensitivity and unfamiliarity with police life earn him, plus others like him, the not so affectionate term, "Doc Nuts."

Do professionals have barriers? Are there white walls? Are officers receiving the professional help that they professionally/ethically have a right to? What is the countertransference toward officers? We quote from Danto in some detail:

> Although psychiatric service was well intentioned and was established to supply the police department in Detroit with help and skilful consultation, the quality of psychiatric service I assessed from the reports contained in the personnel records was almost beyond belief. *Inquiry about feelings* an officer experienced following a shooting remained superficial and there was inaccurate assessment of suicide risk. One of the doctors who gave a police officer approval for return to work and receipt of his firearm, was the same doctor who certified a violent civilian as "not requiring emergency hospitalization" the very day he returned to his community and stabbed his psychiatrist to death. (Earlier that day the patient had pointed a rifle at a window threatening to kill a man inside his home.) There was no follow-up on the officer by the psychiatrists once he had been relieved of his gun, or after it had been returned to him. The reports written by the psychiatrists were entirely administrative and lacked any meaningful interpretation of the officer's problems or practical recommendations. One of the doctors had instructed the officer's wife that he was hopeless and she should leave him. In that manner, *without offering direct help*, the psychiatrist supported the precipitating stress rather than reducing it.
>
> Other officers, whom I have interviewed and treated, have told me that the offices of *some of the psychiatric consultants for troubled officers have a "locked door."* Officers report having been told to *"wait outside,"* only to discover that there is another entrance away from the street entrance at which they are waiting. At this other entrance patients are being admitted while the officer is left standing outside. Or as the officer enters he observes some office personnel who approach him in a friendly manner: many are drinking coffee, but do not offer any to the visiting officer patient. *No greetings of "Hello" or other encouraging remarks are given, and the desk of the psychiatrist is piled high with a collage of reports and papers—all impressing upon the officer that he is "disrupting a busy man's routine."* (p. 38)

What recommendations could be made?

Before we address the many questions raised already—and there will be many more—we return to the question, is there an epidemic of police suicide? The phenomenon has received great attention. The media and Internet are watching. Is there underreporting? Given the stigma, blue walls, possible legal issues, taboo of domestic violence, insurance coverage and the illegacy of suicide, gun control issues, and so on, it should not be surprising. There are cover-ups. There is misinformation. There are, we all know, cases where suicides of police officers are covered up as accidents. This may be for good intentions, but it is also suicidogenic. This does not help our fellow officers at risk! It increases the blue walls. It increases suicides in police.

Although the causal or contributing factors need further study, almost all researchers agree no single explanation will ever be sufficient. Simple findings will add little, except to the walls. There finally has been increasingly more comprehensive investigation. In Canada, the work of Robert Loo (1986) on suicide among the Royal Canadian Mounted Police (RCMP) stands out. Loo studied all deaths during the period of 1960 to 1983. He found 35 suicides; only 1 was female. The annual average suicide rate in the RCMP in the 23-year period was 14.1 per 100,000. There were great fluctuations over the years. All ranks had suicide. Not only among all ranks, but also among job function, years of service, marital status, and sex. Firearms were used by 29 of 35—27 by service revolver, 1 by rifle, and 1 by stabbing. Of the 29 who used firearms, 23 received fatal head wounds. Thus, Loo concluded the rate of suicide in RCMP officers was *lower* than a comparison group from the general population. For example, the RCMP rate was 15.5/100,000, whereas a comparable non-RCMP male in the same age range was 29.4/100,000. Loo thus concluded that there was no epidemic; indeed, he concluded that the rate of suicide among police officers was low.

Why did the suicides in the RCMP occur? Like almost all research, he observed that there was a lack of data. He called for psychological autopsies. (This is a common statement.) Despite the limitations, he found

> There were file entries that suggested a variety of contributing factors to these suicides. As is apparent from the data, . . . most suicides were characterized by multiple factors, of which one might be identified as the key precipitating factor in some cases. The most frequently noted contributing factor to suicide was the distressed psychological state of the member where anxiety and depression were the specific states noted in the documentation. Contributing psychological traits were also grouped here—for example, a member diagnosed as obsessive-compulsive sometime before the suicide. Such traits were typically manifested by a history of personal distress that adversely affected job performance and interpersonal/family relationships.
>
> The second most frequent contributing factor was that of job-related concerns, such as being passed over for promotion, not feeling secure in one's present position/unit, or having to testify before a service or civilian court or commission. In 11 cases, there was evidence of problems in interpersonal relationships with members of the opposite sex, either spouses or girlfriends/boyfriends. In one such case, evidence of this type of problem was well documented in the member's diary and letters.
>
> A history of alcohol abuse or the use of alcohol just before the suicide act, even by members who were infrequent drinkers, was evident in six cases.

> Psychological trauma—for example, the earlier suicide of a family member or close friend, or involvement in a serious motor vehicle accident—was documented in five cases. Financial problems involving debts or the inability to sell one's house were also documented in five cases. Serious illness (e.g., leukemia, heart attacks) was evident in three cases. Of these three cases, two were terminal illness.
>
> It is also notable that 8 of the 35 members were either receiving psychiatric treatment, had received psychiatric treatment in the past, or were recommended for psychiatric treatment. (pp. 384–385)

Loo concluded that suicide is escape. He stated,

> Most of the members appear to have committed suicide in response to life situations that were intolerable (flight from an intolerable situation). Such life situations may also have included an element of grief—that is, the loss of a highly significant factor/person in one's life (e.g., no job promotion, divorce). (p. 385)

Most importantly, Loo concluded that many of the suicides could have been prevented, and he called for psychological/psychiatric services in the police force. He called for police services to have their own psychologist. Police services need comprehensive mental health supports. Much, indeed, can be done to prevent suicide among police.

The rates of suicide in the RCMP from 1984 to 1995 continued to be lower (16.02/100,000) compared with the rate of the general population in Canada. Of course, the question arises whether that is the best comparison group, a perpetual problem (Andrews, 1996a). The stressors often identified in the suicides of the RCMP were alcohol abuse, depression, marital problems, financial difficulties, legal problems unrelated to work, illness, and a family member committing suicide (Andrews, 1996a). Thus, no different from other human beings in general, stress/trauma and a history thereof placed the person at risk. Of course, suicide cannot be simply explained by a trauma (a stimulus); yet at the same time, we must also remember that situational or contextual aspects are always part of the total scenario.

Is it, thus, true that self-inflicted intentional deaths by police is at an epidemic level? Is it increasing? An epidemic, as defined already, is events/incidents of a disease, or psychopathology, or suicide, well above expectations (WHO, 2002). There is a lot of mythology about police suicide (Kamerman, 2001). Violanti (1995), no stranger to the topic of police suicide, suggests, like Danto did, that we do not know. After a comprehensive review of the literature, some have not supported the notion that police suicide rates are abnormally high (Aamoldt & Stalnakar, 2001). Studies on suicide among police show inconsistent results (Berg, Hem, Lau, Loeb, & Ekberg, 2003). Whereas others (e.g., Lynn, 2002) continue to promote the notion of "alarming rates," the question can be asked, Is it an epidemic? To the best of our current understanding, the answer, we believe, is probably, but we do *not* know. Yet much relates to how you make the statement.

What would be a valid comparison group? That is the central criticism about the best study by Marzuk and his team in the United States (Marzuk, Nock, Leon, Portera, & Tardiff, 2002). There was, in fact, a vast array of subsequent editorials to that study. Science calls for comparison; that is, John Stuart Mill's method of difference. This is the critical test. We agree that some suicides are misclassified, yet even taking that into account, our review of the literature would not necessarily suggest an epidemic. At best, we can say that there is police suicide. By the very fact of suicide's multidimensional nature, of course, some officers are at risk, but also so are psychologists, doctors—people. At best we can say suicide rates among police, at least in the Western world, are no higher or lower than *some* comparison groups. It depends on what we are talking about. Finally, there is no need to exaggerate the rate of suicide in police; the tragedy is tragic enough. We, in fact, need to go beyond the question, What is the rate? and ask, What can we do to prevent it?

The main reason Violanti (1995), Danto (1978), Loo (1986), and we offer as the reason for the lack of definitive knowledge is the lack of evidence (facts, in science talk). We do not know because there is a lack of facts (data). Violanti (1995) stated, "Considerable difficulty exists in studying police suicide." Services are reluctant to allow access to such data. They want to keep secrets. The deaths are routinely misclassified as either accidents or undetermined deaths. The myth of "all cops are indestructible" often prevails. There is a "we can take care of our own" attitude.

Police officers are reluctant to seek help. "Officers who feel that they can no longer tolerate psychological pain choose to solve problems themselves through suicide rather than asking for help" (Violanti, 1995, p. 22). There are barriers/walls; there are also the effects, the sting, on survivors. As is true with any suicide, the survivors of a police officer's suicide must cope with police suicide. There is dishonor.

There are many other problems in the study of police suicide (Violanti, 1995). Yet police suicide cannot be ignored any longer. In the past, police services around the world have largely ignored it. However, there is a recent change. This is evident, for example, by the United States's Federal Bureau of Investigation's most insightful document, *Suicide and Law Enforcement* (Sheehan & Warren, 2001). It is a compilation of papers submitted to the FBI Academic, Quantico, Virginia, September 1999. We borrow here and there from that document. (We encourage police officers to consult this report.)

Like many others, including ours, Violanti's solution is to allow for considerable study of police suicide. There needs to be more systematic research.

Fortunately, the study of suicide among police has not only been increasingly allowed, it has become more open. Probably one of the best studies is by Peter Marzuk and his team (Marzuk et al., 2002). We present the study, "Suicide Among New York Police Officers, 1977–1996," but also offer critique of the study. After the study was published, there was a rash of Letters to the Editor in the *American Journal of Psychiatry*. We cite the critiques. We hope in this way to offer the best of all possible empirical knowledge. It also allows us to return to New York City. We can again pose the question: Are police officers today in New York still killing themselves at epidemic levels?

Marzuk and his team examined 668 deaths of police officers from 1977 to 1996: 80 were suicides (12%); the mean age was 33.5 years (the range was 21 to 59); firearms were used in 75 of these (93.8%); the overall suicide rate was 14.9 per 100,000. Is that high? Marzuk concluded, no; he reported that the adjusted suicide rate of a demographically comparable sample of New York City people was 18.3 per 100,000. Thus, Marzuk and colleagues stated, "The police officer suicide rate remained below that of the demographically adjusted rate of the city's population" (p. 2069). They further concluded, "The notion that police are at substantially higher risk of suicide than the average individual may, in part, result from the publicity surrounding a police suicide" (p. 2070).

Of course, even if the suicide rate is low, this should not lull us into a false sense of security. Suicide is a problem among police. Firearms are almost always the method. Easy access and socialization of officers to service firearms understandably contributed to the suicides (Danto, 1978; Friedman, 1967a; Loo, 1986; Marzuk et al., 2002). Marital problems/relationship problems, alcoholism, and job suspensions were highly associated with risk in the more recent New York study, not much different from the 1940s study. Some predictors remain constant over time and place.

Although Marzuk's paper can be seen as one of the best studies on the topic, it has not been without criticism. Next, we offer some criticisms in order to better understand the issues and problems:

1. An inaccurate comparison of police officers with the general population (the general population would include high-risk groups, unemployed, institutionalized, incarcerated, and mentally ill [Violanti, 2004a]).
2. New York City police officers are screened by psychological assessment at the time they are hired: "If we assume that few of the officers [who] committed suicide had a diagnosable preemployment psychopathology, it may not be a fair comparison to look at their rate of suicide compared with residents of New York City generally" (Roth, 2004). The employment screening included the administration of a psychological interview, the gathering of legal, work and relationship histories, a Minnesota Multiphasic Personality Inventory (MMPI), and such. The intent, of course, is to screen out as many high risk candidates as possible. If a similar screening was used with the city comparison group, the city suicide rate would be lower, of course (Dowling & Moynihan, 2004).
3. Since death certificates were used, it is likely that the number of police suicides is underreported (Dowling & Moynihan, 2004).
4. The review of the literature was inadequate; a more comprehensive review would show the rate of suicide in police are inconsistent and inconclusive, namely because of methodological limitations (Hem, Berg, & Ekeberg, 2004).

Marzuk et al.'s reply (2004), elegantly states: We agree, although the "argument could also be made for some homicides." While this may be true, we should not cease our study. "Additional study can help clarify the elements to suicide risk among officers" (Marzuk et al. 2004).

Most studies on police have been done in the United States; greater international comparisons are needed. Yet there are limitations in such comparisons to date; Schmidtke, Fricke, and Lester (2001) reported that the rate of suicide among Federal Police in Germany was lower than a correspondent male, age-matched group (22/100,000 compared with 24/100,000). Thus, rates may vary from the United States and may vary within a country. There is, of course, research on suicide among police worldwide. Lester (1992b) conducted a review of Interpol data on suicide among police for 26 countries. Overall, the rate of suicide was not consistently higher or lower than the suicide rate for men in general in the countries reported. However, rates of suicide among police ranged widely, from 0 (per 100,000 per year) in many countries (e.g., Bahamas, Fiji), to the highest in Luxembourg (75.28 per 100,000). In all countries, firearms were the main method.

Loo (2003) also undertook an international analysis of the suicide rate among police. Using a computerized literature search (Psychlit/Psychinfo and Current Contents), he studied a total sample of 101 police suicide rates worldwide. There were extremes; one suicide rate was as high as 203/100,000. There were great geographic differences. The rates in the American and European countries, for example, were much higher than the Caribbean, Asian, and African countries. There were also differences in the mean suicide rate between different types of police services, such that regional police forces had higher rates than both federal and municipal forces. Loo stated,

> Clearly there is a dearth of useful statistical data published in the open literature on police suicide. Investigators in this field must publish more complete statistics, including breakdowns by demographic variables and suicide rates for comparable groups so comprehensive secondary research can be conducted. Secondary research can draw on existing, even small studies, to perform meta-analyses; identify similarities and differences among different kinds of police forces (e.g., national versus municipal); examine cross-cultural and cross-national differences; examine sex and ethnic differences; and so forth. These types of analyses could address the role of moderator variables such as those suggested in the present study for the role of the presence or absence of psychological services in the police force, social supports, sex, ethnicity, and religion. There is a need to report studies that find no suicide so that the overall picture of police suicide is not inflated by having only studies reporting suicides or, worse, dramatic snap shots that are atypical (i.e., outliers). Several studies have done a thorough job of reporting detailed breakdowns to facilitate meta-analyses. (p. 323)

There needs to be great caution in such cross-national comparisons. As Andrews (1996b) noted,

> Police suicide rates currently available from various nations cannot be directly compared due to differing units of measurement, definition of a police officer, data base used, years examined, sizes of police forces producing widely disparate variability in suicide rates per 100,000, death classification method, and biases to over report/under report. (p. 11)

At best, we can say they vary, thus, calling for much greater agreed-upon systematic study. Maybe the WHO, together with world police services (such as Interpol), can help.

There are obvious gaps in the literature on police suicide. We need, for example, studies into the prediction of police suicide ideation. Violanti (2004b), fortunately, did just such a study. He studied 115 police officers in a northeastern police service in the United States, of which 45 (39.1%) were female and 70 (60.9%) were male. (There were limitations, including the ones listed before when discussing Marzuk's study.) Psychological testing information was protected and not available for analysis. Be that as it may, Violanti found that 27 (23%) officers reported suicidal ideation. The question posed was, Have you ever thought of suicide? Of course, there are limitations to such questions; there are, indeed, great differences in answers, depending on the question asked. Posttraumatic stress disorder (PTSD) was frequently reported. The use of alcohol was very significant. The combination of PTSD and alcohol was reported to be lethal. Further emotional disturbances (psychopathology) were identified. Alcohol abuse has long been characterized as a problem among police; it is a constantly identified malaise in almost all the studies located and read for this book. Violanti (2004b) further concluded, "The rate of comorbid psychiatric and alcoholic disorders significantly exceeds rates that would be expected by chance alone. Lifetime prevalence of mental disorders was found to be nearly twice as high among alcoholics than the general population" (p. 281).

CONCLUDING REMARKS

We need, following the discussion in Chapter 1, research into the cognitive style and logic of police suicidal behavior. For example, what was Lt. Michael Pigott's logic; it must have been something like, "Officers seen by kids, cuffed and jailed, ought to be dead. I am an officer who will be cuffed and jailed. *Therefore*, I ought to be dead." We believe that Michael Pigott must have concluded something like that about the loss of his strong attachment (identification). His need for infavoidance must have, at least, been frustrated—lethally so. Yet his logic meant, "Therefore, it is better to have my children see me in a coffin." That is illogical. What was Michael's actual reasoning? We need to know.

As we reported earlier, psychopathology is a risk factor. Alcoholism is a risk factor. Further study is needed on vulnerabilities (weakened ego). In one unique study of police officers in Norway, Berg et al. (2003) found that suicidal ideation was associated with marital dysfunction, subjective health complaints, weakened ego (reality), anxiety, and depression. Serious suicidal ideation, however, was mainly attributable to personal and family problems. Pionaar, Rothmann, and van de Vijver (2007) reported high rates of suicide ideation among uniformed police officers in South Africa, but also by far, the level was low. Some 92% reported some thoughts of suicide; of course, that rate is the same as in people in general. At least 80% of people think about suicide (Leenaars, 2004). Only 7% had high suicide ideation, however. Again, it depends on the questions asked. Not only the asking, but also what is asked is most relevant. What are we talking about? Little is also known about the incidence of attempts. Berg et al. (2003) reported a lifetime prevalence of 0.7% for attempted suicide. There is an urgent need for such study. We certainly do not know the incidence, for example, in the United States or Canada.

Needless to say, we need to go beyond the individual, beyond the officer's use of alcohol (Did the police suicide abuse alcohol?). The ecological model offers a wider view. We need to understand the relationship, community, and society level. Police culture is paramount. The deaths in New York City in the 1930s teach us that fact. Control is a factor and hopelessness is a factor (Turvey, 1995). Perfectionism is a factor (Slosar, 2001). The situational aspects are important; the environmental factors are important (WHO, 2006). Frequent exposure to stressful situations put police officers at increased risk (Loo, 1984; Maia et al., 2007). Despite the lack of evidence, we know that occupational stress in law enforcement is critical in the suicidal scenario (Loo, 1984). Police women and police families have specific stresses (Loo, 1984). Thus, any consideration of police suicide needs to look at the environmental factors of suicide (WHO, 2006). The World Health Organization, in fact, recognizes that certain vectors in some jobs, like police and doctors, may increase the risk of suicide.

The factors are multidimensional. Suicide among police is a multidetermined event. Yet the most important common criterion, or red flag, of the suicidal police officer is relationship/marital problems (Turvey, 1995). It is a consistent marker to date. We need to understand suicide beyond the individual; the ecological model can guide us. As Kamerman (2001) stated:

> To a great extent, the study of police suicide is dominated by the viewpoint of psychiatrists and psychologists; as a consequence, occupational, organizational and societal factors have tended to be neglected. Suicide in general and police suicide in particular are usually seen as problems whose etiology lies within the psyche of the individual suicide. When factors outside the individual have been taken into account, the almost exclusive focus has been on occupational subculture as it encourages keeping emotional problems to oneself or as it defines the report of suicidal thoughts to the department by fellow officers as a violation of loyalty. But again, the focus is on the suicidal individuals and their comrades and not on large-scale factors such

> as an organization that may be structured to discourage employees from coming forward for help." (p. 530)

Suicide causation is multidimensional, so is suicide-homicide.

Finally, as Danto (1979) argued 30 years ago, if police services are going to reduce suicide among police, police services must learn from suicidology. The reverse is also true. Together, we can better understand suicide in police. If we can understand suicide better, then we can better predict and control it (see Chapter 7). One could want no better in prevention, including to prevent suicide and for that matter, to prevent homicide-suicide.

CHAPTER 5

Homicide-Suicide

The reader will note that the introductory material to each chapter varies in length; this reflects the state of knowledge on the topic. Our knowledge is limited. Before the reader begins this chapter, he should reflect on the rather long introduction to Chapter 1. There we learned suicide is a multidetermined event, so is homicide. Thus, it follows that homicide followed by suicide is also multidetermined. We begin with some reflections from one of the world's best known homicidologists, Nancy Allen. Allen reflected on homicide-suicide, stating, "Murder-suicide offenders are a far less deviant group than the sample of ordinary murders. The majority of murder-suicide cases are married and live in connected family settings, free from criminal associations" (Allen, 1980, p. 86).

These perpetrators are not like killers. They are the everyday officer, not some deviant criminal, but more like suicides. The writings of Marvin Wolfgang, Donald West, and more current authors/researchers are presented along with Allen's. They have all concluded similarly, and we quote Allen again, "All (is) quite different from what is usually implied by the phrase, homicide followed by suicide" (Allen, 1983, p. 165). We need to know more.

Steven Stack, who is the most published sociologist on suicide, has presented the best review on the current research on homicide-suicide. We quote him verbatim, with his kind permission. The genius of Stack is that he not only presents the findings, but also corrects the methodological problem of previous investigations, namely the erroneous and misleading comparison (via J. S. Mill's method of difference) with a homicide group. David Fishbain, Rosemary Barnes (on essential women's issues on this topic), Peter Marzuk, and many other forensic specialists have offered us sufficient understanding, noting unusual findings, but also some commonalities (common factors). Echoing *Othello*, Fishbain concluded some factors learned: "because of the strong affection of the victim, the murder perpetrator did not want to go on living without him or her and committed suicide" (p. 1152). This is called an "identification." The something lost is often a person, but sometimes an ideal, such as not having one's gun removed or not wearing handcuffs in front of one's family. What was the officer's logic to death? Following the discussion in Chapter 1 on logic, we present some thought on whether it was rational or not.

http://dx.doi.org/10.2190/SHSC5

Returning to the topic of sex differences, Fishbain offers one of the best methodological and interesting studies on the topic of homicide-suicide and the only one on female perpetrators of homicide-suicide. He offers some unique facts about women; a revealing read, we believe. He exposes some myths. The main conclusion, like that in males, is that female homicide-suicides are most like suicides. Homicide-suicide is an extension of suicide. There is a continuum, a *stream of violence*. It is suicide. One must wrap one's head around that sole fact to understand homicide-suicide better. Yet the perpetrators are also different than almost all people who die by suicide; they are homicidogenic. A question remains: *On a continuum of suicide, how can one predict a suicidal officer (or any person) also committing homicide-suicide (being a killer too)?*

* * * * * *

INTRODUCTION

Suicide is a multidetermined event. Homicide is a multidetermined event. Thus, it follows that homicide followed by suicide is also not determined by one factor. We cannot here provide all of the literature, but allow us a few signposts. Here is what we have learned about homicide-suicide in the general population. We begin with a direct quote by Nancy Allen (1980), a world expert on homicide and a lifelong friend of Edwin Shneidman. She writes,

> West (1966) has pointed out that murder-suicide offenders are a far less deviant group than the sample of ordinary murderers. The majority of murder-suicide cases are married and live in a conventional family setting, free from criminal associations. The killings are most likely to be of the spouse or child.
>
> The perpetrator commits suicide out of despair rather than hostility. She or he has excessive frustration and enormous guilt because of a greater degree of social consciousness. Selkin's (1976) study revealed that a homicide-suicide usually symbolizes the stark failure of a family's attempt to live together productively. There is evidence of a long-term malignant situation, with either a history of interpersonal discord or a history of life-threatening disease, or both. The perpetrator's attitude toward the victim is marked by ambivalence—jealous rage versus affection so strong the perpetrator removes himself or herself from the murder through suicide.
>
> Freud (1924) noted, "Just as the suicidal person may be attempting to kill an introjected ambivalently regarded other, the murderer may be killing an object of projection; the other, then is one in whom one sees one's own badness. The close linking of suicide and murder is seen in the mechanism of seeing to be killed, to be punished for one's own transgressions particularly for one's own murderous feelings."
>
> In Narioch's (1973) study of homicide in California, it was reported that 10 percent of the perpetrators of homicide commit suicide. This was not found to be the case in the sample this investigator studied. Murder followed by suicide occurred in five percent of the cases studied. Two of these cases

> will be discussed below. These are cases where the suicidal individual had been disturbed by his or her life situation. Both couples were married and living in what appeared to be a conventional family setting as law-abiding citizens. (pp. 86-87)

The early theorists on homicide-suicide were West (1966), Wolfgang (1958), and Allen (1980, 1983) (see Harper & Voigt, 2007). Allen, for example, studied 104 homicide-suicides in Los Angeles during 1970–1979. The rate of homicide-suicides was 2% of all homicides and suicides. However, West (1966) reported a rate of 33% of all homicides and Wolfgang (1958) reported a rate of 4% of all homicides (One has to read carefully; the comparative groups are not always the same). There are further findings of note in Allen's Los Angeles study: 93% of the offenders were male; 80% of the victims were female. (As an unusual tangent, in the West study, 40% of the offenders were female. That is high.) The majority (71%) of the killers were husbands/boyfriends of the victim (2% of the women murdered their children, a subgroup of homicide-suicides. Not all homicide-suicides are the same.) Twenty percent of the victims (4 males and 7 females) and 21% of the offenders (16 males and 1 female) were intoxicated (having a blood alcohol level of 0.10% or higher). Traces of alcohol were found in 29% of the tested victims and 34% of the total offenders. Fifty percent of the victims and murderers had been drinking. Therefore, once more, alcohol increases risk, not only for suicide, but also homicide, and homicide-suicide (Allen, 1980). It can be explosive.

Suicide notes were left by 14% of the homicide-suicides (15 people). We cite an example:

> Dear Mary
> You made it impossible to live with you, and there is no way that I can live without you. I'd rather be dead. I loved you more than life.
> George

This note is prototypical.

Despair appears to be primary. The pain is unbearable. This appears to be more evident than hostility. There is such rage, excessive frustration, and enormous guilt (Allen, 1983). Milroy (1998), however, suggested that after the murder, remorse is a minor reason for the suicide. He asked, "Is it then, revenge?" Our read is that may be true, but also it is *escape*. Indeed, not all homicide-suicides are alike. In one group, there is a history of interpersonal discord, domestic violence, and frequent jealous rage. However, in another group, namely the older or terminally ill, there is an overwhelming sense of incapacitating, painful illness. In another group, often women, there is a history of severe depression, and facing their death, they also kill their children. (Of late, we have also seen the mass murder-suicide, like Harris and Klebold in the Columbine massacre.) Regardless of whether there are one or two or more groups, Allen (1983) concluded that "all (is) quite different from what is usually implied by the phrase, homicide-followed by-suicide."

INVESTIGATIONS OF HOMICIDE-SUICIDE

Steven Stack (1997), a prolific sociologist, has presented the best presentation on the known research on homicide-suicide. He offers the following speculations; we quote verbatim:

CORRELATES OF HOMICIDE-SUICIDE

Most of what is known about homicide-suicide is based on about a dozen, largely qualitative investigations done at the local level. This body of work employs the technique of psychological autopsies (e.g., Selkin, 1976; Rosenbaum, 1990) and the inspection of archival records, such as police reports and psychiatric files (e.g., Boudouris, 1974; Buteau et al., 1993; Easteal, 1994). These data are used to reconstruct the chain of events that led to the homicide-suicide. These studies often involve intense investigations of a small number of cases.

While written from a variety of psychoanalytic, clinical, and psychosocial perspectives, these works have suggested that a number of recurrent patterns typify homicide-suicide. This analysis weaves these patterns into a more coherent whole than does prior work. While these do not fit all cases of homicide-suicide, they appear as dominant patterns in most of the prior research on the United States (e.g., Berman, 1979; Palmer and Humphrey, 1980; Rosenbaum, 1990; Selkin, 1976). The resultant hypothesis largely reflects the main thrust of prior and classic preliminary views of homicide-suicide (e.g., Henry and Short, 1954:117; Wolfgang, 1958).

FRUSTRATED PERSONAL RELATIONSHIP

The genesis of homicide-suicide lies in a frustrated, chaotic, intimate, long-term personal relationship (Berman, 1979; Buteau et al., 1993; Cormier et al., 1971; Danto, 1978; Rosenbaum, 1990; Selkin, 1976; Wolfgang, 1958) and contributes to the risk of violent behavior.

The frustrated, intimate relationship is typically with a spouse or a common-law spouse (Cormier et al., 1971; Rosenbaum, 1990: Wolfgang, 1958). The role of the spouse is typically assumed to be a source of positive attachment, as well as negative affect (Wolfgang, 1958). A high proportion of homicide-suicides involve persons in such relationships. In Los Angeles 71% of homicide victims in homicide-suicides were the wives or girlfriends of the offender (Allen, 1983). Of Selkin's (1976) 13 homicide-suicides, 10 of the victims were the spouse of the offender, the wife in 8 cases and the husband in 2 cases. Palmer and Humphrey (1980) found that 62% of the homicide victims in homicide-suicides in North Carolina were wives compared to only 8% of homicides. In contrast, only 24% of the victims of homicide in homicide-suicides were friends and acquaintances. This number was much larger, 54%, in homicides per se. For an exception to this pattern, see Boudouris (1974).

AMBIVALENCE

A key pattern in the chaotic relationship is extreme ambivalence, a vacillation between anger and love (Berman, 1979; Cormier et al., 1971; Selkin, 1976). The person in this state of ambivalence often feels a dependency on the love object. At the same time, the person experiences a rage at her or him. Persons caught up in this chaos often feel that they cannot live with their love object, but at the same time, they have equally strong feelings that they cannot live without the love object.

JEALOUSY AND MORBID JEALOUSY

That homicide-suicide would be likely to be found in intimate relationships is suggested by qualitative work on morbid jealousy and homicide-suicide. Morbid jealousy is often considered either the most important factor or one of the more salient factors in such chaotic, stormy relationships (Mowat, 1966; Rosenbaum, 1990; West, 1966:82). Morbid jealousy is a delusion, a false idea, that one's sexual partner (e.g., wife, mistress, husband, or lover) has been sexually unfaithful. West (1966) argues that the greatest risk of homicide-suicide rests in men who are paranoid about the perceived infidelity of their love object.

SEPARATION

From the qualitative work on homicide-suicide, the triggering event is often a separation or threatened separation from one's love object. Again, the salience of marital relationship/status is a definitive pattern. A recent separation was found in the case histories of 59% of the homicide-suicides reviewed by Buteau et al. (1993). All of the eight married couples studied by Rosenbaum (1990) were separated at the time of the homicide-suicide. In contrast, only 2 of 24 (8%) couples involved in homicide were separated at the time of the homicide. A study of intimate homicide-suicide in Australia found that 35% of the homicide-suicides occurred after a separation of intimates compared to only 15% of homicides (Easteal, 1994).

DEPRESSION

The offender's separation from his or her significant other is often marked by severe depression, and severe depression is often a key cause of suicide (Lester, 1992). Rosenbaum (1990) found, for example, that 75% of offenders in homicide-suicides were depressed compared to none in a control group of spousal homicides. Buteau et al. (1993) found that 46% of the male homicide-suicide offenders were depressed at the time of the homicide-suicide. Buteau et al.'s (1993) estimate is conservative since it is based on archival records and not supplemented by interviews with the significant others of the deceased. Shepherd (1961) argues that depression combined with paranoid jealousy is perhaps a necessary condition for homicide-suicide.

Using another vocabulary, the combination of rage and depression in the ambivalent offender might be compared to a blend of other-blame and self-blame (Unnithan et al., 1994). While an attribution style typified by extreme self-blame/depression may lead to suicide, and an attribution style based on extreme other-blame/anger may be conducive to homicide, the act of homicide-suicide may require both styles in the offender. The offender may be in a rage given his or her frustration over the separation from the love object. At the same time, given the offender's ambivalence about the relationship, he or she can experience depression as well.

> **HELPLESSNESS**
>
> Selkin (1976) points out that a homicide-suicide may be the only perceived way out of unbearable conflict for the offender. The act is seen as a consequence of unbearable impotence. On the one hand, the offender cannot get his wife/lover back; she is gone. On the other hand, he cannot perceive how he can go on living without her. While the relationship he is in is often basically destructive and at times humiliating, the murderer refuses to give it up (Henry and Short, 1954; Wolfgang, 1958). In carrying out the homicide of his lost intimate object, the offender has the attitude "If I can't have you, no one else can" (Wolfgang, 1958, p. 213).
>
> **GUILT**
>
> The perpetrator's realization that he has committed the crime produces a suicidal impulse. The source of nurturance is lost. The murderer may be overcome by extreme guilt feelings and despair over terminating the source of his nurturance (Buteau et al., 1993; Rosenbaum, 1990; Wolfgang, 1958).
>
> Wolfgang (1958) focuses on provoked guilt as the suicide inducer. In a case of a homicide-suicide in Baltimore, a dazed offender cried out "Oh my god, what did I do?" after murdering his wife (Berman, 1979). Suicide becomes a means for dealing with guilt. Wolfgang (1958:213) cautions, however, that it would be incorrect to conclude that homicide offenders do not feel some of the same guilt as do homicide-suicide offenders. He contends that the difference is one of degree. The homicide-suicide offender simply feels substantially more guilt. He or she has a more well developed superego than the homicide offender.
>
> Psychoanalytic work often conceptualizes the act of suicide as a blend of suicidal and homicidal impulses. Zilboorg (1936) viewed suicide as motivated primarily by spite and revenge. Menninger (1938) contended that suicides tend to be marked by a mixture of homicidal and suicidal motivations. Persons often really want to kill an intimate partner. Instead, they may commit suicide and hope that the partner will feel profound guilt over their suicide. In their suicide notes such persons are sometimes quite blunt and open with such statements as, "Dear ______, you have killed me." On the other hand, suicide is also motivated, in part, by a wish to die, to end a tortured existence. In homicide-suicide, however, both of these motivations are fulfilled. The external object of one's anger is executed. The internal anger one has toward one's self, in turn, is also dealt with violently in a suicide. (pp. 438–441)

The similarities between these observations and the ones that we made earlier on suicide are striking. There may well be a stream of violence. Homicide-suicide and suicide are not polar opposites. They are highly correlated, but also they may be less so to homicide. Homicide-suicide is more a suicide than a homicide. Yet research on homicide-suicide in police, like on police suicide, is lacking. We only located three articles on homicide-suicide in police with the most important published in 2007. However, before we report those findings, we return to the research on homicide-suicide in general.

In his critique of the area, Stack (1997) noted that researchers rarely provided a control or comparison group of homicide and suicide. Samples are often small. There is a lack of systematic analysis, often being only descriptive. There are, thus, a series of methodological problems, and one must remember that critique as we next report a few further studies, to allow us to understand homicide-suicide better.

Stack (1997) studied the records of all homicides in the murder files of the Chicago Police Department from 1965 to 1990. Thus, Stack attempted to correct previous methodological problems by having at least a homicide comparison group. Regrettably, he did not have a suicide comparison group, something commented on by David Fishbain (see below). In the archives, Stack found 267 homicide-suicides. Stack, in his analysis, controlled for sociodemographic variables (possible confounders). For the killers, these variables were male, age, and Caucasian race. For the victims, female, age, and Caucasian race. Statistical procedures, simple bivariate analyses, multivariate and logistic regression analyses, were undertaken representing a sound array of comprehensive statistical techniques.

The incidence of homicide-suicides to homicides in Chicago was 1.65%, low by worldwide standards. Stack (1997) concluded,

> The structural relationship that increases the odds of homicide-suicide the most is that of ex-spouse/lover. For ex-spouses/lovers, the risk of homicide-suicide is 12.68 times higher than in nonintimate homicides. In these cases, the bond that once held a couple together is officially broken. The loss is final; it is no longer just threatened or simply coming in the future. For persons very dependent on the old bond, this loss of their love object can be unbearable. For some ex-spouses/lovers jealousy intensifies after the breakup as they perceive that their former love object is involved with new partners, persons who have taken their place in love.
>
> As anticipated, the current girlfriends or boyfriends of killers are at less risk (6.11 time higher odds of homicide-suicide) than spouses and ex-lovers. Here the bonds are not quite as intense and so the loss of support is not as great. Further, since the couple was not living together, it is less likely that a killer would feel that "I can't live without you" relative to someone he or she is already living with or once did live with under the same roof. (pp. 447–448)

In relation to our previous discussion on Unnithan et al.'s (1994) work on homicide-suicide, Stack (1997) stated,

> This study has some implications for hypothesis formation in the general area of homicide-suicide. Unnithan et al. (1994) have proposed a "stream analogy," wherein the choice between homicide and suicide depends on attributional concerns. Persons and groups faced with frustration will choose suicide to the extent that they attribute the cause of their problem to themselves and to the extent that they are depressed and feel helpless. Other groups and individuals will opt for homicide if they tend to attribute the cause of their

> problem to others and to the extent that they feel angry as opposed to depressed. Drawing on a dozen qualitative studies on homicide-suicide, this study contends that the principal source of frustration in homicide-suicide is a frustrated, chaotic, intimate relationship marked by jealousy and ambivalence. These relationships are marked by a feeling that one cannot live with the other person but cannot live without them either. A separation or threatened separation arouses anger and depression at the same time. The act of homicides overcomes a sense of helplessness. However, the associated depression and guilt over the loss of one's love object result in suicide. Perhaps homicide-suicide can be best thought of as containing both attribution styles discussed by Unnithan et al. (1994, pp. 448–449)

Probably the best Canadian study on the topic is by Jacques Buteau, Alain LeSage and Margaret Kiely (1993), who studied homicide-suicide in Quebec from 1988 to 1990. Buteau and his team examined 39 consecutive cases of homicide-suicide. Sociodemographic data, circumstances surrounding the event, and clinical data were recorded. Yet they noted limitations to the data and called for psychological autopsies. One important homicide-suicide, the case of 14 victims of the mass murder-suicide at the Polytech in Montreal in 1987, had a large impact on the data. These events make a difference. The victims of Columbine would be another extreme example. The thousands of victims of 9/11 make a huge difference. These mass homicide-suicides are different, but also the same (Leenaars & Wenckstern, 2004).

In the Quebec study, the proportion of homicide-suicides to overall homicide rate varied from 9% to 22%. (The proportion to overall suicide rate is not given.) Ninety percent of the offenders were male. The victims, aside from the Polytech victims, were all known to the perpetrator and had been living together as a family or as a couple. Firearms were used in 56% of the cases. Marital discord was identified in 67% of the cases, 56% of the perpetrators had depression, and 23% had substance-abuse problems. Indeed, Buteau et al. concluded, "Homicide-suicide reflects the epidemiology of major psychiatric disorders." This is probably true.

By way of self-critique, Buteau et al. (1993) noted that they did not study suicide. They saw this as a major limitation; indeed, they noted that the data suggest that "Those who commit homicide appear to be different than those who commit homicide-suicide." Further, "homicide-suicide offenders have characteristics similar to suicide-only individuals and dissimilar to homicide-only offenders." This hypothesis is in all probability correct. The offenders of homicide-suicide are more similar to suicide, not homicide.

Buteau and his team further concluded that coroner's files, police reports, and so on, lack rich psychological data. The necessary, unequivocal, evidence is "scarce. This scarcity makes it difficult to offer insightful conclusions. For example, it does not allow us to isolate psychopathology, such as the hypothesis of a high incidence of borderline personality disorder. To date, the research is not sufficient, surely not sufficient to answer the question in our retrospective investigation. They state, "Psychological Autopsies, well known in suicide studies, is the method of choice." The need for psychological autopsies is well recognized (Palermo et al., 1997). We agree.

Fishbain (1994) has also criticized Buteau and his team, namely for the lack of utilization of proper control comparison groups. Fishbain further noted that from his research, presented below, homicide-suicides are more like suicides. This is true about female homicide-suicides. Despite this, the tendency to compare with homicide continues. This is not to say that it is not useful, only that it is lacking. The empirical data call for a comparison with a suicide group or a homicide group and suicide group, but not only with a homicide group. The knowledge from only erroneous comparisons is constricting. Fishbain, Rao, and Aldrich (1985) demonstrated this fact. Thus, caution is in order even about Canada's best study. It has limits.

There are further studies. Felthous et al. (2001), for example, examined the combined homicide-suicide in Galveston County, U.S. from 1980 to 1998. They examined the coroner's office records. They identified 20 killers. Again, the common factors are identified: males are the majority of offenders; guns are a preferred method; domestic violence is present; marital problems and separation occurred frequently before the event; alcoholism was present in most, but not all; and stress was often identified, after the perpetrator was no longer living with the victim or told to leave (although the records did not allow for clear definition of what was meant by stress). There was awareness of another friend/lover. Indeed, like in suicide, a commonality was the troubled interpersonal relationship. A common theme, in fact, was the perpetrator losing or being rejected by the victim. Rejection-aggression is common in suicide, homicide, and thus, homicide-suicide.

Yet once more Felthous et al. noted the psychological information was "disappointingly limited." This has been a pervasive lack; indeed, it is the most commonly cited problem in the studies of homicide-suicides (like in the studies of police suicide). All call for psychological autopsies; we agree that it is the very best method of study (Brent, 1989; Curphy, 1967; Litman, 1984; Selkin, 2005; Shneidman, 1977).

There is, however, one unequivocal fact: intimate partner homicide (and thus, homicide in general) and homicide, followed by suicide, have different characteristics/factors and probably some distinct etiologies. A few differences are the predominance of female victims, the predominance of intimate partner victims, older age of perpetrator, and use of firearm. Lund and Smorodinsky (2001) present a study that examined homicide between intimate partners in California to determine whether homicide followed by suicide differs in important ways from those without a suicide outcome. They studied the homicide files of the State of California during 1996. They found that out of 186 homicides committed by intimate partners, 181 were heterosexual intimate partner relationships. All offenders were male, and 40% (n = 74) committed suicide subsequent to the homicide. The main conclusion was, indeed, that there are significant differences in the characteristics of victims-perpetrators and circumstances of intimate partner homicides and intimate partner homicide followed by suicides. Unequivocally, they are two distinct groups. Lund and Smorodinsky (2001) confirmed the markers (red flags) for the homicide-suicide group: the predominance of males, dysfunctional relations, uses of guns, and so on. Indeed, one of the significant predictors is the use of firearms; it is likely that the perpetrator intended to commit both homicide and suicide by gun to ensure the lethality. Yet once more, these researchers call for more in-depth study.

Rosenbaum (1990), after reviewing the literature and studying 17 cases of homicide-suicide (he studied the files of the Albuquerque Police Dept.), offered depression as a striking difference between people who kill and people who kill, followed by killing themselves. He reported that the large majority of homicide-suicide offenders (75%) suffer from depression; none of the offenders of homicide only suffered from depression. Not only depression, but also other psychopathology is evident (Buteau et al., 1993). The victims differed too. None of the 11 women victims in the murder-suicide group had gross psychopathology; however, most of the victims in the homicide group, both men and women, were characterized by substance abuse, personality disorder, and sociopathy. Not only the perpetrator, but also the victim in homicide-suicides are different from homicides. Rosenbaum concluded,

> The findings from the present study suggest that patients with the following features may be at risk for murder-suicide: depression, male gender, and married or living with a woman in a long-term relationship characterized by discord, physical abuse, and frequent separations and reunions. Furthermore, men at risk for murder-suicide are likely to abuse alcohol, have a history of violent behavior and previous depressive episodes, and have a longstanding personality disorder. The most important feature is the presence of morbid jealousy. West said, "The greatest risk of murder-suicide would occur in paranoids . . . especially those in whom the emotional distress takes a depressive form" (West, 1966, p. 81).
>
> The onset of the depression is associated with the breakup of the relationship when the woman leaves. The tragedy is triggered when she tells the man that she is leaving for good or that she has a lover. The final confrontation with severe verbal and physical violence, often abetted by alcohol, then explosively erupts in murder, which is quickly followed by suicide. From a psychodynamic point of view, the depression may be viewed as a defense against the underlying aggressive and murderous impulses. However, if the "trigger" incident produces intense enough aggressive impulses, the depressive defense is breached and the "murderous impulse" is released. The perpetrator's immediate realization that he or she has committed the crime leads to intense guilt, return of the depressive defense, and suicide. (pp. 1038–1039)

Suicide as aggression turned inward has been presented; it is a well-accepted fact. However, the intense role of aggression in homicide-suicide appears to be equally critical, but also not well known. It is cited in most police cases. As one homicide-suicide perpetrator said, "If I can't have you, no one can." This is common, aberrant thinking, a lethal major premise. It easily follows, "I can't have you. Therefore, no one will. I'll kill you."

We would be remiss if we did not highlight the importance of domestic violence in homicide-suicide. It is present in almost all cases (Bossarte, Simon, & Barker, 2007). It may well be universal (at least common), and we address the concept further elsewhere. Of course, domestic murder-suicide is the ultimate example of domestic violence. The fact that it is almost always a male phenomenon needs to be better understood. Why is it that men, in particular, are so determined not to allow their partners to leave? Why would the male offender feel jealousy and hatred to such extent that they would rather kill the one they love and die themselves than to accept that their partner no longer wishes to be part of their lives? Like others, Barnes (2007) suggests that these are urgent women's issues. From the ecological model of violence, there are social circumstances of homicide-suicide. Barnes (2007) suggests power/control is central. She offers a feminist perspective and "argued that the patriarchal nature of our society provides the fertile context for the individual to kill a loved one and then commit suicide" (p. 10). (This is true in the police culture.) If so, we need to look to the ecological model for effective, comprehensive intervention.

The discussion to date begets a core issue: What about female homicide-suicide offenders? Regrettably, there is only one study; yet it is probably one of the best-designed studies of the topic, a study by David Fishbain and his team (Fishbain, Rao, & Aldrich, 1985). We will, in concluding this section on homicide-suicide, examine their study in detail. Maybe it will allow us to understand homicide-suicide in females better.

Making the now obvious observation, female homicide-suicide perpetrators are rare and unusual (Fishbain et al., 1985). The percentage of female to all homicide-suicides has been low. Further, given that homicide-suicides are more like suicides, there had been no study until Fishbain on the very topic. Fishbain and his team examined the case files of the Dade County Medical Examiners Department from 1957 to 1981. Inclusion in the homicide-suicide group was determined by the principles of medicolegal death (coroner) investigations, albeit they have limits. Control groups were selected; female homicide victims in homicide-suicides were compared with female homicide perpetrators in homicide-suicides and with female individual suicides. Thus, there are three groups. The information reviewed was as follows: death certificate, report of the police officer investigating the deaths, medical examiner's autopsy report, toxicology report, suicide note if written, newspaper clippings, hospital records if patient lived for a while after the homicide or suicide, and previous hospital records if available. All available chart information was reviewed for all three-victim groups. The task was a very large undertaking, but also most helpful, including to us.

Of 133 homicide-suicides identified, 10 cases were perpetrated by females (7.5%). Significant differences were found between the groups; yet the female homicide-suicide perpetrators were more like female individual suicides than female homicide-suicide victims. The following were the results:

The following items were determined to be significantly different between female homicide-suicide perpetrators and female homicide-suicide victims: type of residence, living with whom, object of homicide, type of discovery, weekend deaths, presence of suicide note, and recent history of depression.

The following items were determined to be significantly different between female homicide-suicide perpetrators and female individual suicides: type of residence, living with whom, and recent history of depression.

There are a great number of relevant facts. The majority of homicides involved family members or acquaintances; this is even more so for murder-suicide. It is largely a dyadic event. There is a strong attachment (identification). "Typically," stated Fishbain et al., "because of the strong affection of the victim, the murder perpetrator did not want to go on living without him or her and committed suicide" (p. 1152). This was true for Othello and probably many police perpetrators. After the homicide, suicide becomes escape. Female perpetrators were much less likely to live with the spouse or acquaintance than female homicide-suicide victims. The object of the homicide, compared with male perpetrators, was much more likely to be a lover or ex-lover. There was an extreme and probably dysfunctional intimacy providing a primary source of attachment; once this is lost, jealous rage may occur (Selkin, 2005). Often the discovery of the homicide-suicide was not a surprise to survivors; yet in female homicide-suicide perpetrators, it was almost always not anticipated. No one knew or predicted it. Few people expected the tragedy; no one knew who the perpetrator was. There is deep isolation. Is masking/dissembling more common in female homicide-suicide perpetrators?

Compared with data on male homicide-suicide offenders, female homicide-suicide perpetrators are less impulsive, and more planned the murder. For example, they more often leave a suicide note. These women's murders are not impulsive, but are intentional. There is a high degree of preplanning, in fact. This is opposite of the common lore about female perpetrators being seen as only victims, who impulsively kill the partner and then themselves in response to chronic domestic violence. We are not suggesting that does not occur, but Fishbain allows us to see these women differently.

Alcohol, although present, was not discriminative. The weapon was usually a gun, but also it does not discriminate.

On one more important point, the female murderers in homicide, followed by suicide, often saw themselves as acting in self-defense, but also the suicide followed nevertheless. It is likely that despite trauma, such as domestic violence or loss, the female perpetrators felt remorse or guilt. Suicide became an escape. Female perpetrators had abusive, unstable relationships. They sometimes killed their partner while being beaten, sometimes in self-defense, but not always. The murder was sometimes victim-precipitated. Of course, the question arises, is this true in a specific case?

Female homicide offenders frequently suffer from mental disorder, notably affective disorders and alcoholism. Personality disorders are often evident. However, female homicide-suicide perpetrators differ. Female homicide-suicide perpetrators more often suffer from depression. Thus, the female homicide-suicide offenders are quite different from female homicide perpetrators and female homicide-suicide victims. Yet Fishbain et al., show that they are more like female individual suicides. There are, in fact, very few statistical differences. Thus, Fishbain concluded that female homicide-suicide can be best understood as types of suicide, not as homicides. We agree.

Mental disorder (psychopathology) is a striking similarity between suicide and homicide-suicide. Female individual suicides are most likely to have a history of depression than female homicide-suicide perpetrators, who in turn are more likely to have a history of depression than female homicide-suicide victims. The percentages are as follows: 92% versus 40% versus 2%. Suicide and psychopathology, or an inability to adjust, are intimately related. The same is true for homicide-suicides. Psychopathology is a risk factor.

The main conclusion from this sole study on female homicide-suicide is that they are most like suicides. Homicide-suicide is an extension of suicide (Marzuk, Tardiff, & Hirsch, 1992; Milroy, 1998).

Let us cite one more study: Barraclough and Harris (2002) studied all homicide-suicides in England and Wales from 1988 to 1992, and consistent with other research, found that the act is "a family matter," with predominantly men killing their current or past wife, followed by girlfriend, common-law wife, ex-girlfriend, and ex-wife. A few go on to kill their children too. Only a few men kill strangers. Women, if they committed murder followed by suicide, typically kill the children. They note, from this first national study of England and Wales, the following: "Notably rare are instances of women killing adults and then themselves." They found one out of 161 incidents, a 0.6% rate, who killed her husband. There were 18 other female perpetrators (n = 19, 15% of total) and they killed their children. This is a common act in female homicide-suicide perpetrators worldwide. Women in England often kill their children, followed by suicide, not their lover, husband, and so on.

Yet Fishbain (2003) noted that there might be great cultural differences. For example, the incidence of female perpetrators is higher in England than the United States. In a U.S. sample (Fishbain et al., 1985), out of 133 homicide-suicides, 10 (7.5%) were female perpetrators. In all the cases in this sample, the victim was of the opposite sex (60% were lovers/ex-lovers.) Therefore, Fishbain concluded that not only the incidence, but also the characteristics/dynamics of homicide-suicide may be different in men and women and also in different cultures. He argued, and we agree, for much greater systematic study. We need to know more not only about males but also about female homicide-suicide perpetrators. Overall, there is little in the literature on female perpetrators.

CONCLUDING REMARKS

Suicide of a loved one has often been considered a suicide risk factor. This appears to be true for homicide-suicide too (Perdue & Brookhart, 1974). There may be a contagion. Goldney (1979) described a case where a woman, two days after the suicide of her husband, assisted in her children's death and then killed herself. He presents the following facts of the case:

> **Medical Responsibility in Murder and Suicide**
>
> The recent report from the United States of a woman encouraging her children to jump to their death, and then doing so herself, two days after the suicide of her husband, should not be passed off merely as an aberration of the American scene. From the psychiatric point of view, such a tragedy provides a salutary illustration of some of the clinical features evident both in the uncommon *folie à deux* (or, in this case, the *folie à famille*) situation, and in cases of family murder followed by suicide.
>
> It would appear that the husband, who allegedly had a schizophrenic illness, had been the dominant member of the family, even to the extent of convincing other members that he was the God of a new religious sect. That his family shared these delusions was evident from the writings of his children in which reference was made to their belief that their father was God. That such beliefs could persist, not only in the wife, but in children up to the age of fourteen, was due partly to their singularly vulnerable personalities, but also to their isolated existence in hotels, with virtually no contact with the outside world and, therefore, little opportunity for reality testing.
>
> It is of note that the suicide of the husband was not followed by the restoration of equilibrium in this family, and presumably delusional thinking persisted. This emphasizes the fact that mere separation from the primarily ill person may not be sufficient treatment in the *folie à deux* situation.
>
> It is difficult to avoid the connotation of murder of the children by the mother before her suicide, even though it is reported that some of the children were apparently willing enough victims. One can surmise the fantasies of mother and children wishing to be reunited with their dead husband and father, and it is such fantasies which are of particularly grave prognostic significance in the management of suicidal patients. (p. 50)

A question remains: On a continuum of suicide, how can one predict a suicidal person (or officer) not only dying by suicide, but also committing homicide-suicide?

CHAPTER 6

Homicide-Suicide. Police

This will be the second briefest interstitial section, simply because there is very little known about homicide-suicide among police. There is one sole nomothetic (general) study, *ONE*. This is the study by, to now no stranger to the field, John Violanti. One could want no better authority.

Suicidal individuals are profoundly aggressive. Homicide-suicide in police is so. Violanti's study offers some very first insights. The number-one conclusion: *homicide-suicide in police is not low*; it is much higher than in a sound comparison group, the general population (again, via Mill's method of difference). Is it at an epidemic level?

Violanti presents an array of multidetermined information, many the same as suicide or homicide-suicide. One of the major determinants of police suicide is relationship problems. Is domestic violence highly implicated? There are unbearable problems, frustrated needs, many workplace stresses, and regressive strains. Is alcohol use often a precursor? Are there blue walls? Are guns almost always the lethal weapon? Does the service revolver availability increase risk?

Thus, we are left with a high incidence of homicide-suicide in police, but little has been studied or done. Violanti's study is very rare. Would they do the same if there were a high incidence of cholera or SARS among police? Like so many before, Violanti and we call for study. We need to know what we are talking about. What are we investigating? Only then can we treat it effectively, which we will look at next.

This chapter is concluded with a definition of homicide-suicide, one applicable to police.

* * * * * *

INTRODUCTION

Suicidal individuals are profoundly aggressive. Homicide-suicide in police is so. Violanti (2007) stated,

> The perpetrator is unable to accept the failure of what he thought was a satisfactory relationship. The perpetrator is viewed as an aggressive individual who hides behind a façade of self-assertion, is unable to withstand the

http://dx.doi.org/10.2190/SHSC6

> reality of an unexpected rejection, and possibly a drastic life change. He commits suicide after killing his extended self. (p. 97)

Although homicide-suicide has a low base rate, it has a profound effect on a police officer's family, friends, community, and the police service. Homicide(s)-suicide, of course, do occur among police offenders. They are rare events; however, a unique and new study by John Violanti (2007) offers some of the same insights as 1940.

The established incidence of domestic violence among police officers is high, significantly higher than the general population. Police officers appear to be at high risk for homicide-suicide, probably higher than the general population. Domestic violence appears to be heavily implicated in police homicide-suicides. One of the major determinants of police suicide is relationship problems; there are unresolved problems, frustrated needs, stresses, and regressive strains. Yet this is the case for many suicides too. Domestic violence is often a precursor. Alcohol use is often a precursor. Yet despite the facts, there has been no study until 2007. Why? Is it the walls?

Violanti's (2007) method is important; he writes,

> Data on police homicide-suicides was collected from police_dv@yahoo groups.com, a website devoted to topics concerning domestic violence and related problems in police families. Accounts of police homicide-suicides were extracted from newspaper accounts of the incidents described on the website. A sample of 29 homicide-suicide cases were collected, ranging from January 1, 2003 to February 28, 2007. There were several newspaper articles on each incident, providing increased robustness of information for the present study. While some may question the validity of newspaper reports, Rainey and Runyan (1992) point out that newspapers are a viable source of information for intentional injury surveillance. They found that newspaper reports were decidedly more complete for variables of interest than reports filed with governmental officials in the area of the event, and have potential value in raising public awareness. (p. 100)

Violanti concluded that homicide-suicides among police are *high*. He identified 29 cases; it is not as rare as many believed. Everyone will be in disbelief. Survivors, officers, and many others did not believe a homicide-suicide could happen among officers. It appears, however, that it is not that rare. Violanti further cautioned that homicide-suicide in police is increasing. The majority of victims were women (n = 24, 83%); however, five of the victims were men killed by women police officer offenders. (This would suggest that homicide-suicide in female officers is much higher than the general population.) The primary weapon was the service revolver (90%). Table 1, copied from Violanti, presents the descriptive characteristics of the police homicide-suicides sample.

Most incidents occur at a local police department level (76%), as opposed to state or national levels, echoing the observation by Loo on police suicide. Yet many facts, due to the source of information, were not available. For example, the use of alcohol could not be determined. Thus, much greater study is needed. Will the police services finally allow for such, given the epidemic level of homicide-suicide in police?

Violanti also does the helpful thing of presenting cases; we present one of his below.

> A 33-year-old Police Deputy Inspector shot his 28-year-old wife several times, killing her. It happened on Friday night during an argument the couple had in their car. The officer had earlier approached his wife in a cafeteria and ordered her into the car. He later committed suicide. During the month prior to the homicide, the wife told friends she felt threatened and afraid. However she never filed any claims or notified the police. He was well-known as a campaigner against domestic violence, only weeks earlier receiving praise for his efforts in the protection of women. (p. 101)

It is often the individual (idiographic) that gives us the greatest insights (Allport, 1942, 1962). This is in police homicide-suicide. Of course, there are cautions in case presentations. Yet some conclusions can be made. Violanti stated an obvious one: "The key to prevention of homicide-suicide may thus lie with reduction of domestic violence." Again, although this is not always the case, it is generally so. We agree that domestic violence prevention is a key, but suicide prevention may be even more so a key.

Violanti concluded:

> Difficulty in the internal detection of police domestic violence exists for other reasons. Many victims will not report domestic violence incidents to authorities because of shame, guilt, or fear of reprisal. As one police spouse stated, "You don't anger your husband when he carries a gun." In reported incidents, police administrators may not take complaints seriously. They may not fully understand the dynamics of domestic violence and thus may fail to take proper action. Other supervisors may believe ignored domestic violence problems will solve themselves. (Violanti, 2001)

Recent passage of the federal Domestic Violence Gun Ban Law prohibits persons convicted of domestic violence offenses from owning or using firearms. While the law intends to decrease the risk of injury or death, it may also add to obstructing detection of police domestic violence. Officers will increasingly hesitate to report other officers for domestic violence because such officers will have their firearms taken away and will likely lose their jobs. Chief John W. Lamb, head of the Denver Police Department's Civil Liability Bureau, succinctly stated,

> The police department has no unarmed positions, so if this law is not changed, it will be career ending for those affected by it. If you can't carry a gun, you can't do your job. (cited in Clark, 1997, p. 103)

Not only to save lives, but also to address legal issues, this is paramount. Selkin (2005) presents a case of homicide-suicide in a police officer. He states,

Table 1. Descriptive Characteristics of the Police Homicide-Suicide Sample (n = 29)

	n = 29	(%)[b]
Homicide Victim		
Year of occurrence		
2003	1	3.4
2005	7	24.1
2006	15	51.7
2007[a]	3	10.3
Age of victim		
7–30 hours	8	38
31–40 years	9	42
41–56 years	4	15
Gender of victim		
Male	5	17
Female	24	83
Relationship to perpetrator		
Wife/ex-wife	16	55
Girlfriend/ex-girlfriend	8	28
Child	3	11
Husband	2	6
Homicide-Suicide Perpetrator		
Age of perpetrator		
24–35 years	6	35
36–40 years	6	35
41–57 years	5	30
Gender of perpetrator		
Male	27	93
Female	2	7
Weapon used		
Service firearm	26	90
Other	2	10
Rank level		
Patrol officer	15	52
higher rank	14	48
Type of department		
Local	22	76
State	6	21
Federal	1	3

Table 1. (Cont'd.)

	n	(%)[b]
Circumstances		
Motivation for act		
Divorce/estrangement	10	35
Domestic violence	12	42
Marital problems	2	7
Other	1	4
Presence of domestic violence		
Yes	18	62
No	11	38
Past domestic violence		
Yes	20	70
No	9	30

[a]As of February 2007.
[b]Percent does not add up to 100% due to missing cases

> A 43-year-old police officer, distraught upon learning that his wife was going to divorce him, took his service revolver and murdered her, their two young children, and then took his own life. Surviving close relatives, two stepsons, sued the community where the tragedy had occurred claiming that the police department had not responded appropriately to earlier calls for help on the 911 call placed by the murdered woman. The police response a year earlier when Officer Murillo had physically abused his wife was inappropriate, and in violation of department policy. By failing to arrest Murillo on that occasion, the officer defendants enabled him to retain his job as police officer, and remain in possession of his weapon. Murillo was never confronted with his dangerous behavior and required to accept responsibility for his actions. A number of other significant but subsidiary allegations were made in the suit. (p. 81)

Pam (2001), in her FBI paper (Sheehan & Warren, 2001), made the same observation on the relation of police homicide-suicide to domestic violence. She presents two incidents:

> Officer Patrick Fitzgerald, a patrolman in the New York City Police Department (NYPD), shot and killed himself, his wife and their two small children in their family home in September 1998. One month later, a veteran Newark, New Jersey, police officer, Heriberto Gonzalez, murdered his girlfriend—a rookie police officer—and then committed suicide. Both incidents involved prior histories of domestic violence; examples such as these are proliferating all over the country. (p. 358)

Suicide is murder turned 180 degrees. Suicide is violence turned inward. Suicide and homicide are two sides of the same coin. Similarly, depression and anger are interwoven. (There are strong biological correlates.) People who are depressed, as we discussed earlier, are at risk for suicide. They may feel unbearable pain, hopeless, helpless, and so on. The same is true for people who kill someone, followed by dying by suicide.

Homicide and suicide, as we discussed, are both acts of violence, lethal violence—other-directed or self-directed, but violence nonetheless. Homicide-suicide is violence, both other- and self-directed. Pam (2001) writes,

> Homicide and suicide as separate acts are different from homicide-suicide as a combined act—suggesting that a new synergy is in play when these behaviors are bundled together. It is my view that those who commit suicide after committing murder do so not because they are clinically depressed but for reasons rooted in concerns and perceptions about the altered shape of their posthomicide world. This might include grief over the prospect of living without the victims or love objects, fear of disgrace, scandal, humiliation, financial ruin, stigma, demotion, job or career loss, drop in status, arrest, incarceration, hospitalization, etc. In short, such depressions appear to be more situational than existential, fruits of an acute, albeit self-generated crisis—the consequences of which are intolerable, less bearable even than self-inflicted oblivion. While clinically depressed suicides distort and color data and are unable to imagine the future, homicide-suicides seem to intuit and assess their now-altered future all too realistically and guided by their personal value system and circumstances, pragmatically choose death as their most acceptable option, solution, or mode of escape. Accordingly, it would be the aggressive, not the depressive, part of their personality that drives the suicide *and* the homicide. If true, this would constitute a critical difference among the groups. (p. 359)

Police homicide-suicide, a subset of police suicide (Pam, 2001) is receiving ever-increasing public and media attention. Yet there has been a lack in the professional, scientific literature, both forensic and mental health. Why? Like others, Pam suggests, in part, this has to do with the police culture of guns. Pam states,

> Only recently have we begun to recognize that American police officers who engage or have engaged in certain behaviors, especially domestic violence, should not possess guns.
>
> This point of view is especially embodied in the Lautenberg Amendment, a federal law signed on September 30, 1996, which amended the Gun Control Act of 1996, making it unlawful for any person convicted of a "misdemeanor crime of domestic violence" to possess a firearm. Currently facing constitutional challenges in District Court of the District of Columbia, the Lautenberg Amendment makes it probable that officers who lose their guns will also lose their jobs. Domestic violence advocates are heartened by this new legal weapon, viewing it as an important step in protecting

> intimate partners of police officers, police families and the police officers themselves. (p. 361)

Would gun control help? There is no question that gun control reduces suicide and homicide (Leenaars, 2007). However, what are realistic gun controls for police? Although the author is a lead researcher in gun control in Canada, we do not advocate the removal of all guns from police. We believe, in fact, that that would be lethal in the Unites States and Canada. That is different, however, than removing a gun from an officer at risk for suicide or homicide, whether in the United States or Canada. Indeed, it is the law!

On another note, dissembling/masking is not rare. Police who are about to kill other or self are generally concealing. There is intention. They do not want anyone to know their plans, often well preplanned in female perpetrators, it seems.

Pam, thus stated,

> Because those planning to commit suicide will generally conceal their intentions, no current test, instrument, clinical technique, screening method, or biological marker can conclusively predict suicide, much less murder-suicide; but there *are* clues. The potential for murder-suicide might include acute indications of hopelessness and obsessive preoccupations involving "jealousy, paranoia and fantasies of reunion or deliverance and salvation during episodes of major depression, postpartum depression, or psychosis (often bipolar). (p. 362)

What can be done? Pam concluded the following at the FBI conference on police suicide:

> Because of job-related variables and personality factors, police officers appear to be disproportionately at risk for suicide and its subset, homicide-suicide, compared to other occupational groups. They have access to guns, which some use as instruments of violence against others or themselves, usually with lethal results. Domestic violence appears to be heavily implicated in police murder-suicide, a situation that the Lautenberg Amendment seeks to address by permanently barring any officer ever convicted of the misdemeanor of domestic violence from possessing a firearm. There does, however, continue to be institutional denial about the role of police stress and frequency of abuse in police families, the latter variously estimated at 25–40%. Officers who do not separate the streets from the home employ interpersonal traits, skills and coping mechanisms rewarded on the job but inappropriate to interpersonal relationships. Moreover, police culture and training encourage control, aggression, authoritarianism, domination, a strong sense of entitlement and other conduct that correlates with batterer behavior.
>
> The synergy of a murder-suicide combination makes it distinguishable from individual homicide or suicide, although each behavior shares some common risks and potentiating factors, especially aggression/impulsivity, stress, access to weapons and if concurrent, alcohol/substance abuse. While it is impossible to conclusively predict suicide or homicide-suicide, there are

> clues and indicators that make interventions possible. In all events, law enforcement supervisors should be vigilant in order to circumvent behaviors by police officers that harm others as well as themselves. (p. 363)

Pam may be correct, but Fishbain's study of female homicide-suicide perpetrators would suggest that homicide-suicide is more like suicide than homicide. Indeed, it is a suicide.

CONCLUDING REMARKS

To conclude, thus, we now know that homicide-suicide in a police officer can be defined as

> Currently in the Western world, homicide-suicide is a conscious act of other and self-induced annihilation, best understood as a multidimensional event in a needful individual who defines an issue for which the homicide, followed by the suicide, is perceived as the best solution.

CHAPTER 7

Suicide. Homicide-Suicide. Police: Prevention

Karl Menninger taught that "The patient is always right." Much of our treatment of suicidal officers is figuring out how they are right, even if they wear a blue mask (dissembling). The way to understand how the officer is right is in the natural progression from understanding to application to practice. Once one knows the officer, then treatment comes naturally.

The proof of suicide *prevention* is in the "ventions"—as in prevention, intervention, and postvention. We are here most focused on intervention, specifically *psychotherapy*, and in the final chapter, we will again address some reflections and recommendations in all the "ventions." The main payoff of all our research and training activities—which we hope includes both on the street and in this book—lies primarily in making our efforts more effective. That is what counts in the psychotherapy room. In the first section of this chapter, we repeat some ideas from the research, namely from the work of Edwin Shneidman, Michael Lambert, Lester Luborsky, Bruce Wampold, and Dan Rudofossi (specifically on officers with a prevailing mood disturbance, PTSD). We hope to show some of the special aspects of psychotherapy with suicidal officers, based on our evidence-based theoretical understanding—both the general and the unique—of the suicidal police officer. They will cast some new light. We begin with the question, Can police prevent suicide among police?

The first section of the chapter outlines the application of our theory for crisis intervention and for psychotherapy, both officer-centered, with police. It is the core of what we have learned to be useful and life saving in the psychotherapy room with officers.

Ann-Marie Berg, a well-respected European expert on our topic, has clearly established that the main obstacle to help-seeking in officers is the negative attitude toward such. There are enormous blue walls. What are these blue walls? Are they different than in the 1930s? Why has this remained the main obstacle?

The fact: a multimodal or multicomponent approach is needed to help suicidal and homicidal-suicidal officers. Medication, hospitalization, and gun control may be needed, which we will explore.

http://dx.doi.org/10.2190/SHSC7

Ultimately, the question remains: Are all police officers helped by psychotherapy or environmental control or whatever? Are some officers never helped? Why? We offer some unique thoughts on the topic by Herb Hendin, and Harvard's current most famous suicidologist, John Maltsberger. The number one error: No communication. Every officer can resonate to that one.

This chapter, we hope, will allow one to progress from conceptualization to understanding and then move to what we can do to prevent the events. We have to be person-centered or officer-centered. Ultimately, no psychotherapy with suicidal officers can be isolated: Our treatment may involve the family, friends, fellow officers, minister, family doctor—all of us, not only the psychologist or psychiatrist. It takes the community. Suicide prevention in our fellow officers is everyone's business, every officer's business.

* * * * * *

INTRODUCTION

Can police prevent suicide among police? Can police homicide-suicide be prevented? What can we do? We will next briefly address the topic of prevention, most specifically, intervention.

Suicide among police occurs; yet some in the media (Horvitz, 1994) reported, "Cops kill themselves at three times the rate (of the general population)." This may be a myth. Having said that, officers do kill themselves. The reasons for suicide in police are complex and often elusive (Horvitz, 1994). We hope that the reader of this book has learned something. We need to know what it is that we are preventing.

One of the most common notions in policing is that officers should handle their own problems. There are barriers (blue walls). There is dissembling or masking. Often, the attitude is to "take care of their own" (Barrett, 1997). There is a stigma. Sometimes suicides are classified as accidents or undetermined. The classical study in New York already revealed that fact, never mind the negative impact on survivors. They suffer so after; there are skeletons, a sting. Horvitz (1994), in a review on the topic states,

> The culture of the police force reinforces the notion that officers should handle their problems on their own. "Some men take it as a sign of weakness to go for help," Suaci says, "It's important to get the message across that it's really a sign of strength." As Ivanoff views it, "The officers have been taught from day one of their training that they have to be in control, they have to think of other people. The missing component in training is when to call for backup personally.
>
> Resistance to seeking help often is grounded in fear of repercussions. Of the 11 police officers who committed suicide this year in New York, only one was being treated by an NYPD psychologist at the time of his death. Officers believe they may be stigmatized if they admit they have a problem. "If I indicate that I need help, they may take away my shield or

> weapon and put me behind a desk and I'll be labelled a psycho," says Shaughnessy, describing the worst-case scenario. In other jobs, employees usually have no way of knowing that a coworker is receiving counselling. However, in the police force, Mancuso says, "Everyone knows as soon as the officer's firearm is removed that he's receiving counseling—it's instantaneous." (p. 11)

A common view is that police officers possess negative attitudes toward seeking professional help. However, there is a lack of empirical study (Berg, Hem, Lau, & Ekeberg, 2006). A nationwide study in Norway (Berg et al., 2006) studied police officers' use of professional help compared with the general Norwegian population (something that Mill's method of difference, as you have read, called for in science). They found that, although officers were inclined to seek help from family doctors, few contacted psychologists or psychiatrists. Only 10% of officers contacted psychiatrists or psychologists, even by those reporting serious problems with anxiety and depression, and even serious suicide risk. Few sought help, and if they did, it was solely for medication. The strongest association with help from a psychiatrist or psychologist was, in fact, solely for medication, not for psychotherapy or counselling. Age was not a factor. Years on the force were not a factor. Sex was; female officers often sought help more than male officers. Thus empirically, police officers are, indeed, likely reluctant to seek professional and, at times, life-saving help. There are blue walls.

The blue walls are high. Police officers may dissemble; they may live behind a façade, not letting his true self be known (Barrett, 1997). What can we do? Of course, the walls are not only attributable to the officers. Their superiors also may be blamed. The walls are not only high, but also complex. Officers are sometimes sent to psychiatric/psychological services as a form of punishment. We need to overcome this. This is a serious risk factor for suicide (as we read earlier in this book), and probably for homicide-suicide in police. Indeed, police services need to recognize an obligation to deliver help to officers (Barrett, 1997; Horvitz, 1994). Some police services have done little to address the problem, making officers make statements like, "Is anyone listening?" (Barrett, 1997). Fortunately, there are many police services today that do so. We believe that the mental health system also helps; yet there is more that can be done. We address this issue further in the recommendations.

Police are our current knights. In police culture, they may have to be macho. Officers often subscribe to the macho myth (Barrett, 1997). Yet police often experience trauma, stresses, and such more so than the public. They see homicides, pain, and the like on a daily basis. They also see suicide and homicide-suicide in their own. That is trauma. In addition, there is the gun; they have lethal means. It is a symbol of power—of life and death. They hold the trigger. Thus, we need to shatter the myths about suicide, homicide-suicide, and their prevention.

CONFIDENTIALITY

Before we address intervention, we need to make one more point regarding confidentiality. Experience and research show that officers are reluctant to see psychologists, social workers, or psychiatrists. Some fear that what they say in therapy will not be protected (Powers, 1999). Confidentiality is a legitimate issue in intervention.

We here offer some guidance from Powers (1999) and the Chicago Police Service. They state,

> **Privilege and Confidentiality**
>
> Privilege is a right held by the individual in counselling that prevents confidential information from being released in a court of law or other legal proceedings without permission of that person, unless so ordered by a judge after a hearing.
>
> Confidentiality refers to the obligation of a therapist not to disclose information about their client to anyone unless permission has been granted by that person. Together, these two principles greatly restrict what a therapist can release about a person in counseling.
>
> **Are Police Officers Protected?**
>
> The Chicago Police Department's Professional Counseling Service, St. Michael's House, psychologists, psychiatrists and social workers are obligated and required not to disclose any information about a police officer in therapy or counseling. Once a professional relationship has been entered into with any therapist, confidentiality is automatically imposed. However, the exceptions to confidentiality listed below apply to the aforementioned services and/or persons.
>
> **Limitations Placed on Protections**
>
> In general, there are four situations in which all therapists are required to break confidentiality.
>
> The first is suicide. If a counselor believes that their client is going to kill themselves, they are obligated to do everything possible to ensure that a suicide does not occur.
>
> Second, if a client indicates that they are planning to harm another person, the counselor must attempt to notify that individual of the threat.
>
> Third, if a client relates that they have engaged in or are presently engaging in child abuse, the therapist must immediately notify the Department of Children and Family Services.
>
> Fourth, if a client sues a therapist for malpractice, therapists have the right to defend their actions and this defense may include releasing notes from therapy sessions.
>
> **Are All Department Programs Protected?**
>
> No. The only Department unit mandated to adhere to the strict rules of confidentiality is the Professional Counseling Service. Other units, or Department programs such as the Behavioral Intervention System, Personnel Concerns Program and the Fitness for Duty/Psychological Evaluation System

are not covered by rules of confidentiality. The reasons that these programs are not covered are two-fold. First, they do not create a professional, therapeutic relationship with the employee. (As noted above, a professional relationship is required before a person can assume that confidentiality exists.) Second, these programs are *non-disciplinary, management based* and were designed to address issues of work performance and/or fitness for duty. Though these programs are not covered by confidentiality, access to private files is restricted. It is important to realize, however, that this restriction of access to files is not the same as confidentiality.

Conclusion

Counseling and therapy cannot work without an atmosphere of trust. The foundation of trust is confidentiality. The Professional Counseling Service, counselors from St. Michael's House, as well as most therapists in private practice, must adhere to the code and ethics of confidentiality.

What can we do? What can we do about suicide? Homicide-suicide?

TRAUMATIZED POLICE OFFICER-PATIENTS

September 11, 2001; the four RCMP officers killed in Mayerthorpe, AB; the suicide of Lt. Michael Pigott in New York; the four officers in the "homicides-suicide by cop" in Oakland, CA; the homicide-suicide of fellow officers in London, ON; and so on, are traumatic events. They are outside the range of normal human experience, even for police officers and other public-safety and security personnel. Officers are more frequently traumatized than the general public, not only by one event but also continually. By the very nature of their job, officers of blue, red, and white experience ongoing trauma throughout their career. Administration is at high risk. For many, it is not one event, but many. Ask anyone who went to the World Trade Center after the collapse. (We have many friends who did so.) We need to not only understand Posttraumatic Stress Disorder (PTSD) in officers, but also to offer clinicians a guide to complex PTSD syndrome in officers and public safety professionals (Rudofossi, 2006).

PTSD is not rare, of course. PTSD is a normal (not crazy, mental, or whatever) response in a person exposed to a traumatic event in which both the following are present:

1. the person experienced, witnessed, or was confronted with an event or events that involved actual or threatened death or serious injury, or a threat to the physical integrity of self or others
2. the person's response involved intense fear, helplessness, or horror (DSM-IV).

Traumatic events would "horrify, repulse, disgust, and infuriate any sane person" (Rudofossi, 2006). Rudofossi, a psychologist-police officer, being well aware of this, asks the now obvious question, "Why shouldn't that be true for police officers?" Regrettably, after traumatic experiences, a common response is, "Snap out of it," or "Don't talk about it," or "Just get over it" or "Go on with your duties." Many officers do not; indeed, this avoidance only exacerbates the problem. Many do so; yet forgetting, avoidance, phobias, and inhibition, as was first well-documented in survivors of PTSD in Vietnam veterans, only traumatizes the officer more. We need to break down the blue wall of silence. The loss or trauma, all too often, result in becoming "disenfranchised"; the core loss that officers experience. She is then caught in the no-win cycle of persistently reexperiencing the event (such as recurrent and intrusive distressing recollections, recurrent disturbing dreams, acting as if the event was reoccurring) and persistent avoidance (such as efforts to avoid activities, duties, having an affair; leaving the force; restricting affect), with increased symptoms of difficulty falling asleep, irritability, difficulty concentrating, hypervigilance or startle response. In addition, in some, even suicide or homicide occurs. Yet there is hope; despite taboos ("You have to be the tough guy"), clinicians, psychiatrists, and psychologists can help. An officer's ability to adjust to a trauma is largely affected by the type of response provided. The critical issue is, Is the environment supportive or not? Rudofossi shows us how to be supportive, not only to the officer but also to mental health professionals as well. He offers a unique guide to healing, and thus, better policing.

To illustrate, on March 3, 2005, in Mayerthorpe, Alberta, James Roszko killed four RCMP officers: Constables Anthony Gordon, Leo Johnston, Brock Myrol and Peter Shiemann. Not only were those murders traumatic, there were aftershocks. Officer Jeff Whipple, along with Officer Jim Martin narrowly escaped being killed by Roszko. Only because of a call from an investigator into the Roszko case, were they delayed. They were first to arrive at the murder scene. Officer Jeff Whipple has stated that the scene was traumatizing; he reported that he suffered "significant nervous shock and emotional suffering." Whipple continued to be traumatized, he now reports (Ex-officer Sues Over Mayerthorpe, 2009), as he provided services to relatives of the slain officers. Interviews and discussions with investigators resulted in Officer Whipple reexperiencing the trauma over and over. He reported that he suffered shock, but that nothing was done. Officer Whipple did not receive professional help nor, he claimed, was offered such. His mental health, as one would predict from a PTSD diagnosis, deteriorated. Officer Jeff Wipple recurrently reexperienced the event that involved horrific actual deaths and a threat to his physical integrity. He responded with intense fear, helplessness, and horror. By September 2008, he was permanently disabled and was no longer employed as an RCMP officer. Nothing had been done. Officer Wipple was not alone; Officer Allen Starman has also claimed that the aftermath traumatized him and, despite suffering overwhelming shock, he was forced to continue being involved in the investigation (Second Mayerthorpe Officer Sues RCMP, 2009). He asked for help and a transfer, but he was denied. Understandably, he suffered mental health problems, likely PTSD, and was medically discharged in 2007. Wipple and Starman were not alone! They suffered a normal health response to common police trauma, but the blue walls in all probability caused pain and an emotional disorder, PTSD, or some other adjustment disorder. Regrettably, this occurs all to often among police, including after suicide among police. Is there hope for Officer Jeff Whipple?

What about the sting of the "horror," in the words of Acting Chief Howard Jordan, of Saturday, March 21, 2009, in Oakland, California? Officers Mark Dunikan, John Hege, Erv Romans, and Dan Sakal were killed in a suicide by cop incident. The trauma did not end there. The aftershocks were not only for family and relatives, but also fellow officers. The sting continued; will it? Jordan acknowledged that it was " a very emotional day." He stated that officers "are all feeling the same pain, rookies and veterans alike, regardless of assignment." Will the blue culture finally offer hope in Oakland now? Or will it be more of the same?

The first step toward hope for officers in Oakland, London, and elsewhere is for them to seek help. Psychotherapy is needed. A working alliance needs to be developed in therapy; the therapeutic relationship between officer and doctor will be critical. Clinicians need to understand the officer; effective treatment is based on being person-centered (oriented) or officer-centered (oriented) (Leenaars, 2004). What would it be like for Officer Whipple? You have to know whom you are treating. Clinicians need to know who officers are. Empathy and officer-therapist goal consensus are essential. A collaborative-based approach is needed; yet all need to get beyond the blue wall (officer), and white wall (therapist). We all have our myths. We need to not only break the walls, such as, "It's just a matter of fact—Standard Operating Procedure (SOP)," but also we need to lessen and prevent the aftershocks, the unbearable pain, not only for the officer but also for her family—and sometimes for the whole department. How does a department cope with the deaths of fellow officers?

To quote, Rudofossi:

> Casting the glow of our own private dreams as human beings without mediocrity, apologetics, or being patronizing is one of the liberating gifts that may be shared. By sharing some of our hopefully optimistic positive myths through self-disclosure as a model for our officer-patients to choose, modify, or reject in their public or private myths, clinicians as public and private service professionals offer a priceless gift as well. Clinicians can also learn a great deal through the fascinating resilience and insights police and public-safety officers offer through their lens of experience as pilots of their safety and ours as well. They must remain our number one priority! To paraphrase Hillel, "If not by us, by whom? If not now, when?

PSYCHOTHERAPY WITH SUICIDAL OFFICERS

Suicidal people need psychotherapy. Psychotherapy has a long history (Freedheim, 1992). The intent of therapy with suicidal people is to reduce the person's psychological pain. To quote Edwin Shneidman (2001):

> If the villain is psychological pain then we need something that fights that pain. There is a word for that: *anodyne*. An anodyne is a substance that (or an agent or person who) assuages pain. Psychotherapy in general ought to be anodynic. But with a highly suicidal patient—with *perturbation* and, even more seriously, high *lethality*—the anodynic function of the therapist is vital. (p. 182)

Our method with our suicidal patient is to serve as an anodynic agent "to relieve the pain so that the patient's *raison d'être* for suicide is mollified and the need to end the inner suffering is no longer pressing" (Shneidman, 2001, p. 182).

Effective psychotherapy should be person-centered—or patient-oriented (Task Force on Empirically Supported Therapy Relationships, 2001). Person-centered or police officer-centered psychotherapy is derived from the focus on the individual—the individual in his (ecological) entirety; that is, biological, psychological, sociological, and so on. It follows the ecological model. This is why it is also sometimes called multicomponent or multimodal psychotherapy. This simply means that it is not only psychotherapy alone—cognitive-behavioral, interpersonal, psychoanalytic, dialectical behavioral, whatever—that is most useful, but it may be even more effective in some cases in combination with medication, and removing the gun from the officer may be even more effective (Leenaars, 2006).

The core question is, Is psychotherapy effective? Can it reduce police suicide?

Psychotherapy research is well established today (Strupp & Howard, 1992). The empirical answer to the question can be found in Michael Lambert's 5th edition (2004) of Bergin and Garfield's classic in the field of research, *Handbook of Psychotherapy and Behavior Change* (see also Garfield & Bergin, 1978). What psychotherapy is, thus, effective? Freud (1916/1974) was at pains to differentiate his psychotherapy from others; the *modus operandi* of psychoanalytic psychotherapy was to be unique (Strupp & Howard, 1992). The claim to superiority has been made—Beck, Ellis, Rogers, Wolpe, to name a few. Yet to quote Strupp and Howard (1992), "The seeming uniqueness of each system might simply be semantic or stylistic or reflect previous fashions" (p. 313). The view is "that common factors may be of overriding importance in all forms of psychotherapy" (Strupp & Howard, 1992, p. 313). A systematic review (Leenaars, in press) showed that there is no *superior* psychotherapy for suicidal people, in fact. Many psychotherapies are effective.

The issue, Is psychotherapy effective? is like asking, Is surgery effective? A better question would be Bruce Wampold's (1997): "Which treatments are most efficacious for which patients under which conditions?" (p. 21). Or, which treatments are most effective for which officers under what conditions?

To return to Wampold's (1997) common factors, he writes,

> The features that are shared by all therapies included in a single study are designated as common features. The most ubiquitous common feature of therapies is the therapeutic relationship and consequently, for all imaginable studies of psychotherapy, all treatments would involve the therapist and

> the patient forming a relationship, making this a common feature. Sensitive and empathic responding to patient-expressed pain could likely be a common feature. (p. 26)

The importance of the therapeutic relationship has received more attention than any other common factor in psychotherapy (Lambert, 2004; Lambert & Bergin, 1992). Perhaps the most influential early study on the topic was a paper by Luborsky, McLellan, Woody, O'Brien, and Auerbach (1985). Luborsky and his colleagues begin with the obvious fact to most practitioners: there is wide variation in the effectiveness of individual therapists. They reported a study of the differential outcomes of patients seen by different therapists.

Luborsky's main conclusion was the now obvious: Patient therapist relationship is an important predictor of outcome for psychotherapy. Luborsky et al. (1985) first concludes,

> Our first finding of wide differences in therapist effectiveness by itself has potentially important implications for the study of psychotherapy. In particular, it is now widely accepted after decades of comparative studies that although most forms of psychotherapy are demonstrably effective, there have been little evidence for significant differences in outcomes among different psychotherapies. (p. 609)

Luborsky further concluded,

1. Therapist personal qualities have exerted their main influence on the therapist's ability to form helping therapeutic alliances.
2. The therapist's ability to form rapport or an alliance is possibly the most crucial determinant of the therapist's effectiveness.
3. Once a therapeutic alliance is established, the therapists who persistently do what they are supposed to do are most effective.
4. The qualities that are required to treat a person effectively can be used with other people—including suicidal people, of course.

The American Psychiatric Associations' practice guidelines for assessment and management of suicidal patients supported the view that the therapeutic relationship is central (American Psychiatric Association, 2003). What are the qualities of an effective therapeutic alliance? Are there commonalities with suicidal patients?

THERAPEUTIC RELATION WITH SUICIDAL PATIENTS

As previously stated, we hold to the tenet that understanding is a key to prediction and control. If we know the lethal suicidal officer, we can treat him effectively; or the converse, if we do not, we cannot treat him effectively. This is consistent with Shneidman's challenge: "We ought to know what we are treating." To answer the question of the therapeutic relationship with suicidal people, let me begin with some discussions in November 2001 in Edwin Shneidman's home (Shneidman, 1981a, 1984, 1985; see Leenaars, 1999a). The author asked on that occasion whether he had any thoughts about psychotherapy with suicidal people. He offered:

> Suicide prevention is about a person, a person wanting to be helped to stop their pain, what I call psychache.
>
> In a sense, suicide prevention tries to mollify the whole person. Psychotherapy is concerned with what kind of person that individual is. What works is a view held by Sigmund Freud, William James, Erwin Stengel, not Pavlov or Skinner or any reductionist view.
>
> Our kind of treatment, psychotherapy and so on should address the person's story, his/her narrative, not the demographic, nosological category or this or that fact. It says, "Please tell me who you are . . . what hurts?" Not, "Please fill out this form . . . and give me samples of your body fluids."
>
> Of course, the practical disadvantage of this approach is that it requires more than a few minutes per patient. Suicide prevention is not an efficiency operation. It is a human exchange.

Suicide prevention is based on a humanitarian approach to life, not what Danto (1978) observed in the 1970s. White walls do not help. The psychotherapy that works with suicidal people is a person-centered therapy, or if you prefer, an officer-centered therapy. There is research to support the claim that the relationship (attachment) that the therapist develops is central in effective psychotherapy with suicidal patients. Donaldson, Spirito, and Overholser (2003), for example, presented a study with a group of suicidal people receiving a cognitive-behavioral mode (a specific task-oriented treatment) and the other suicidal group receiving a nondirective mode. What these researchers learned is that it did not matter what treatment the patients received. Patients in both groups showed positive response. Thus, this study replicated Luborsky et al.'s (1985) finding with suicidal patients. It was hypothesized that the relationship was critical. Suicidal people were telling their narratives and someone was listening (after all, these patients were important; they were part of a research study). Keep in mind in this study, the same seven therapists did both treatments; maybe they were just good therapists. Psychotherapy is the attachment, not simply this or that technique. What works is mollifying that person's pain. What works is quality care.

One further study on the relationship being so important with suicidal people is worth noting. Wasserman (2001), in a longitudinal follow-up study, found that suicidal patients with multiple contacts with different people over years had a much higher rate of suicide than expected. They were the suicidal patients that had most frequently been seen by different people over time, after various attempts. These people, in fact, received the not-too-unusual practice, when people find their way to clinics or hospitals. They are never assigned to *the* doctor, nurse, therapist, and so on. According to Wasserman (2001), these suicidal people never received the attachment that they needed to traverse their pain. They remain detached and escape.

"Suicidal people," says Shneidman, "need a human exchange." This is not armchair speculation, but evidence-based practice. A task force of the American Psychological Association (APA) Division of Psychotherapy, Division 29 (Task Force on Empirically Supported Therapy Relationships, 2001) identified the following common elements of effective therapy relationships: therapeutic alliance (or rapport), therapist empathy, and patient-therapist goal consensus and collaboration.

Lambert and Bergin (1992) agree; they cite some of the core conditions as empathy, worth, and positive regard. The list may seem like one from Carl Rogers (1951), but behavior therapists too have embraced concepts such as warm, sensitive, and the like (Lazarus, 1971), and so have cognitive-behavioral therapists (Beck 1976; Beck & Freeman, 1990; Meichenbaum, 2005). Lambert and Bergin (1992) stress these ingredients as essential means to establish rapport. Luborsky et al. (1985) stated the same; they use such descriptions as "supportive," "liked very much by the patients," "very persistent in trying to help." Yet they also highlight APA's Division of Psychotherapy finding on goal consensus and collaboration. Luborsky et al. found that those therapists whose sessions contained the highest adherence to the goal(s) of treatment showed better performance in the cases. They called it the purity of the therapy. They write,

> The high correlation between purity of technique and patient outcome suggests that once a helping alliance is formed, the therapists who do what they are supposed to do achieve their effectiveness in this way. However, an equally tenable, reverse-direction interpretation is that when a patient experiences a helping alliance, he enables the therapist to adhere to his intended technique. (p. 610)

There should be goal consensus and collaboration, regardless of therapist dimensions or officer dimensions. The goal with suicidal officers is often obvious: Keep the person alive.

OFFICER/PATIENT QUALITIES

What about patient qualities? Of course, our very first premise on patient qualities, including being suicidal, is Shneidman's dictum: We ought to know what we are treating. And this implies in a person-centered approach: We ought to know *whom* we are treating!

Beyond this dictum for success, research has shown that the patient's attributes contribute to the process and quality of the therapeutic relationship and the outcome of the treatment (Lambert & Bergin, 1992). Of greatest concern are the variables that might correlate with negative change (Bergin & Lambert, 1978) and even death (Hendin, Haas, Maltsberger, Szanto, & Rabinowicz, 2004). The more severely disturbed, troubled, and so on most suicidal patients are, the greater the probability of negative results. Patients diagnosed with schizophrenia and borderline personality are difficult in psychotherapy in general (Bergin & Lambert, 1978). This is probably true with such patients if suicidal. However, equally important are interpersonal factors; Kernberg (1973), for example, reported that low quality of interpersonal relationships (lack of rapport) was a poor prognostic sign. Yalom and Lieberman (1971) found that low involvement in treatment resulted in little effect of the treatment. (Blue walls would cause such.) Lambert (2004), in his review of the more current research, supports this view: No relationship, no treatment.

Why do patients leave psychotherapy? This is an equally complex question. Jerome Frank's classical work is often associated with this question (Lambert, 2004). Frank, Gliedman, Imber, Nash, and Stone (1957), for example, asked the question and identified many reasons for why people leave psychotherapy, but one of the best markers is the lack of *perseverance*. Perseverance is "the habit of seeing things through despite obstacles that would be expected to be relevant to remaining in psychotherapy, which is a long term task, requiring considerable tolerance for frustration" (Frank et al., 1957, p. 295). This is, of course, the stimulus for suicide: intolerable frustration: PAIN. Will the suicidal officer persevere? What will help? Can the police officer be mindful, accept the unacceptable, and so on? Can he accept being cuffed and jailed? Can she accept the loss/rejection of her boyfriend? Can he cope with his gambling debt? It is of interest that this characteristic is relatively independent of what task or demand the person faces in life. Edwin Shneidman's advice on this topic was "The trick to life is not to spoil and ruin it, no matter what happens."

THERAPIST VARIABLES

Under this heading, therapist qualities could be an endless list of factors (Beutler et al., 2004; Lambert, 2004). The research, in fact, has long shown that there is considerable consensus in studies that ask the patient what was most helpful; they will state the therapist (Lambert & Bergin, 1992). Some therapists are more effective than others (Luborsky et al., 1985). There are, of course, factors that are harmful; some deteriorate the process (Hadley & Strupp, 1976; Lambert, 2004) and some that are suicidogenic (Leenaars, 2004; Leenaars et al., 2002).

EFFECTIVENESS

Maybe it is appropriate to leave the question, "Is psychotherapy effective?" last, although the topic has been embedded throughout this discussion. Psychotherapy is effective in helping people achieve their goal and overcome their psychopathology, even suicide risk (Lambert & Bergin, 1992). This is faster than natural healing, leaving the person alone, and the like. Of course, every psychotherapy has not been studied with every patient or every police officer. Be that as it may, the average psychotherapy patient is better off than 80% of untreated people (Lambert & Bergin, 1992; Smith, Glass, & Miller, 1980).

The question of how much therapy is enough is important, for both practical and theoretical reasons. Some espouse 12 sessions, but research shows that most patients would be underserved (Lambert & Ogles, 2004). Lambert and Ogles, in fact, write,

> Research suggests that a sizable portion of patients reliably improve after 10 sessions and that 75% of patients will meet more rigorous criteria for success after about 50 sessions of treatment. Limiting treatment sessions to less than 20 will mean that about 50% of patients will not achieve a substantial benefit from therapy. (pp. 156–157)

Are all police officers helped by psychotherapy? Or are some officers not helped? Are there negative consequences? The literature is scant, and there is nothing on suicidal police officers in psychotherapy that do not benefit (Lambert & Bergin, 1992; Lambert & Ogles, 2004). Two variables that have been associated with negative outcomes in patients in psychotherapy in general are more severe problems and significant interpersonal difficulties. The percentage of negative consequences may be as high as 5% (Lambert & Ogles, 2004), but then this is true with medication, hospitalization, or any treatment. Much greater research is needed, which may help in identifying those patients who benefit and those who do not.

What is ineffective? Are there common problems in psychotherapy with suicidal patients? This may well be one of the most important questions, namely because they can—and have—resulted in deaths by suicide. There is only one, a most unique study on the question, the work of Hendin et al. (2006). They examined the cases of patients who died by suicide while receiving psychotherapy (and most also medication and some hospitalization too). Therapists of 36 patients were studied by multiple methods. Hendin and his group isolated six recurrent problems: poor communication between therapists, permitting patients and their relatives to control the therapy, avoidance of issues related to sexuality, ineffective or coercive actions resulting from the therapist's anxiety, not recognizing the meanings of patients' communications, and untreated or undertreated symptoms. It is important that all therapists, regardless of orientation, pay very careful attention to these *common* problems, and not only in psychotherapy with suicidal people.

MULTIMODAL OR MULTICOMPONENT APPROACH

As we learned, some patients are difficult to treat with many suicidal patients being an obvious example. The research suggests that with such patients, one must be multimodal (or multicomponent) (Lambert, Bergin & Garfield, 2004; Leenaars, Maltsberger, & Neimeyer, 1994). This simply implies that to treat a lethal suicidal person, one may have to use adjuncts to psychotherapy. Psychotherapy with suicidal people often requires a multimodal (or *ecological*) approach (Thase & Jindal, 2004). Active outreach and use of community resources (e.g., telephone crisis lines) are integral to psychotherapy with almost all suicidal people. Psychotherapy with highly suicidal police officers should be a community approach. Coordination and collaborative involvement of others, such as family members, nurses, social workers, clergy, and so on are, in fact, strongly supported by the American Psychiatric Association (2003). It is a guideline to treating many suicidal people effectively; indeed, it was part of the guidelines at the very beginning of modern thought about effective treatment of suicidal people (Shneidman & Farberow, 1957). Medication, hospitalization, and direct environmental control, such as gun control may be effective interventions and can be life saving. Gun control may act as an anodyne (Leenaars, 2007, 2009b). However, given that medication may be life saving for many, we next briefly discuss it. We will then turn to one of the most effective strategies in violence prevention, environmental control (see WHO, 2006, *Preventing Disease Through Healthy Environments,* a document on which the author consulted).

MEDICATION

Psychotherapy and medication are effective and often necessary to prevent suicide (Bronisch, Wolfersdorf, & Leenaars, 2005; Möller, 2001; Slaby, 1994; Stahl, 2000; Verkes & Cowen, 2000). The combination of the two may be lifesaving. Yet like psychotherapy, there is no specific somatic treatment of suicidality (Möller, 2001). There is no antisuicide pill.

It is assumed that effective psychopharmacological treatment lessens the risk of suicide, although it has been difficult to demonstrate this (Verkes & Cowen, 2000). This echoes the problem on effective psychotherapy. What medication works? Which ones are effective? What medications are effective for which person? It is beyond the scope of this book to address these questions, but for example, it is known that there are essential links between suicide and depression. Up to 60% of suicidal people suffer from a mood disorder, although this is lower in some countries, ethnic groups, and so on. There is strong support for the belief that some suicides have a serotonin dysfunction (Asberg et al., 1976; Maltsberger, 2002), but that is not the only brain dysfunction.

In depression, there is heightened perturbation. The pain or anguish is unbearable. Mental pain fuels the jump into the suicidal abyss. It is an accepted fact that the depressed state of many suicidal people is related to serotonin dysfunction in the brain. Thus, drugs that are specific serotonin receptor inhibitors can be most effective. The selective serotonin re-uptake inhibitors (SSRIs) "have revolutionized the outpatient treatment of depression" (Maltsberger, 2002, p. 86). Best practice would dictate that many—not all—depressed suicidal people could be effectively treated with the SSRIs. Yet equally, good practice would dictate that this treatment be combined with psychotherapy. Maltsberger (2002) concluded,

> I continue to believe that psychotherapy in the treatment of suicidal patients remains extremely important, and that it often makes the difference between living and dying. The newer antidepressants, however, now are an essential part of the treatment of most depressions of any severity. Psychotherapy combined with antidepressant drugs is often the best treatment for the patients. (p. 87)

Maltsberger's view is shared by many (for example, Hollon & Fawcett, 2001). Yet there are cautions. "For a very small vulnerable subpopulation SSRI drugs may provoke suicidal states" (Maltsberger, 2002, p.86). However, this is true about many medications, not only SSRIs.

In psychopharmacology, are there unique vulnerable individuals who have reactions to otherwise comparatively innocuous drugs? Paul Hoch (1972) stated,

> Acute reactions can occur in certain persons following a single dose of one or more types of drugs or intoxicants . . . one must be aware that even a single dose, in predisposed individuals, is capable of occasionally provoking an acute organic reaction. (p. 160)

In psychopharmacology, like in psychotherapy, we have to be person-centered. One must also evaluate risk of the availability of medication, just like availability of the service revolver (Leenaars et al., 2009). What is life saving for many, may not be so for that police officer (Thase & Jindal, 2004). Of course, some suicidal officers may need even greater multimodal intervention; for example, hospitalization and environmental control.

ENVIRONMENTAL CONTROL

As we learned in Chapter 1, Shneidman (1985) has continually asserted that there are no universals in suicide, only commonalities, and we would add homicide-suicide to that classification. It is a suicide, not homicide, but then so is suicide by cop. Both are not homicides per se, but suicides. Yet there may be one universal truth in the prevention and that is: Gun control works.

One area with prevailing consensus that a public health approach can be effective, in fact, in suicide prevention has been means restriction (Leenaars et al., 2009; WHO, 2002, 2006). Erwin Stengel (1964) was one of the first in the last century to propose a public health approach as a means for decreasing the incidence of suicide. For example, he noted that the detoxification of domestic gas (from coal gas with high carbon monoxide content to natural gas) might have reduced the suicide rates in nations where the switch had taken place.

Subsequent research on the detoxification of domestic gas in England supported Stengel's proposal. A comprehensive review of the research around the globe supports the approach more generally, often called controlling the environment (Leenaars et al., 2000). After careful analysis of all measures by an international team of researchers, headed by Bertolote (1993), a series of tactics to prevent suicide supported by the empirical literature were proposed. Among the tactics were gun possession control, detoxification of domestic gas, detoxification of car emission, and control of toxic substance availability (Leenaars et al., 2009). Medication control is essential. Among the WHO list, gun control legislation is often cited as the prototypical example of public health intervention to prevent suicide (Bertolote, 1993; Leenaars, 2009b; WHO, 2006). Gun control is an excellent example because guns are a lethal method and easy availability, like for a police officer, obviously can facilitate death. One would predict that availability would increase suicide and that stricter gun laws would reduce the suicide rate. There are ample laws, for example, in Australia, Canada, New Zealand, and the United States to allow for scientific investigation. We will briefly review the research on the association of the availability of the means, guns, and suicide, and on the effect of gun control legislation or laws on suicide.

From a public health perspective, one can study the association between firearms and suicide at the individual level and population level, sometimes called the ecological level. Each has limitations, but also benefits. The problem with the individual (case-control) empirical study is finding reasonable controls and allowing for generalization, often from small groups, to different groups. The problem with the population studies includes the "ecological fallacy," drawing conclusions about individuals from groups (aggregate) data. (We already discussed this in the preface.) Each has its strengths, and together, we can generalize to both the individual *and* population.

The availability of guns is difficult to measure, and often only indirect measures are available—the accidental death rate by firearms and the percentage of firearms used for crimes such as murder (Lester, 2000). There are, however, a few studies on actual firearm ownership, such as measured by gun licenses, but none in the police. In the United States, measures of actual firearm ownership are available in nine geographical regions (but not by the 48 states) Markush and Bertolucci (1984) found that in the United States, actual ownership was positively associated with suicide rate by shooting and total suicide rate. Lester (1988b) replicated the finding that ownership was positively associated with the firearm suicide rate. Lester (1988c) found that ownership of firearms in Australia was positively associated with suicide by shooting; Carrington and Moyer (1994a, 1994b) reported that firearm suicide was associated with ownership in Canada; and Etzersdorfer, Kapusta, and Sonneck (2006) concluded the same in Austria. Therefore, it is well established that there is a strong positive correlation of firearm suicide to the rate of gun ownership. For police, availability of a means makes a difference and thus, the next question arose: Would restriction of the means reduce suicides (and violence in general)? (Leenaars, 2009b; Leenaars et al., 2000).

INDIVIDUAL LEVEL STUDIES ON GUNS AND SUICIDE

At the individual level of empirical studies, the findings "indicate that a gun in the home is significantly associated with a higher risk of suicide, especially among the young" (Miller & Hemenwey, 1999, p. 73). Kellerman et al. (1992), in a frequently cited study, found that people who died by suicide were more likely to have a gun in the home. During 32 months, they studied all cases of suicide that occurred in the home of the suicide in two urban areas, Shelby County, Tennessee and King County, Washington. They controlled for sex, race, age range, and confounding variables (such as failure to graduate high school, living alone, consumption of alcohol, current medication, hospitalization). After controlling for the confounders, the presence of a gun was highly significant. The risk was higher when the gun was a handgun, loaded, and kept in unlocked storage. Not only study of overall age groups, but also the study by David Brent (Brent et al., 1993) on adolescents has shown the same fact.

On a different tactic, but also very relevant to environmental control, the research at the individual level showed that the association between guns and suicide is not simplistic; there are a host of relevant factors. Psychopathology and drug/alcohol abuse, especially alcohol, are associated in the complex equation (Miller & Hemenway, 1999). If a suicidal person has an emotional disturbance, a gun in that home greatly increases the risk for suicide. Furthermore, the results of an individual (case-control) study of the associations between guns in the home and homicide show the same findings (Cummings et al., 1997).

POPULATION LEVEL STUDY ON GUNS AND SUICIDE: GUN CONTROL LAWS IN CANADA

Although countries differ in the most frequent method of suicide, firearms are a preferred method in some countries. This is true in Canada, for example. Gun control, by strict licensing and restricted availability of firearms, is often cited as the prototypical example of public health intervention to prevent suicide (Bertolote, 1993).

An opportunity for studying the effects of legislative means restriction (e.g., gun control laws) on their use for suicide is provided by Canada's Criminal Law Amendment Act of 1977 (Bill C-51), enforced since 1978. This Act required acquisition certification for all firearms, restricted the availability of some types of firearms to certain types of individuals, set up procedures for handling and storing firearms, required permits for those selling firearms, and increased the sentences for firearm offenses.

Early commentators on the Act (Mundt, 1990) reported little impact of the Act on firearm suicide in Canada, but presented only simple charts, with no statistical analysis of the trends. Lester and Leenaars (1993, 1994) conducted a comprehensive study on the preventive effect on suicide of the Act in Canada. The results suggested that strict firearm control laws may have been associated with changes in suicide rates due to the reduced use of firearms for suicide, and no overall switching from firearms to other methods for suicide. Lester and Leenaars' results suggest that Bill C-51 in Canada appeared to have had a significant positive impact; namely, lowering the rate of suicide by guns.

Subsequently, Leenaars and Lester (1997a) examined whether the restriction of firearms in Bill C-51 in Canada had a preventive impact for those of all ages or only for some ages. The results showed that the percentage of suicides using firearms decreased only for those aged 15 to 64, while it increased for those aged 65+. Thus, the general conclusion seems to be that the impact of making the gun control laws stricter in Canada on suicide was not apparent in those over the age of 65, but significantly so in the young. Shneidman and Farberow (1957) had already shown that the suicidal elderly have a stronger intent to die than younger adults. They are less ambivalent and there is a chronic course to the death (Leenaars, 2004). Younger suicides, and this would be true for younger officers, are more situationally disturbed and mentally constricted (Leenaars, 2004). Perhaps the younger officer may be sufficiently delayed by increased difficulty in obtaining the preferred method for suicide so that the suicidal pain has passed by the time that he has succeeded in obtaining the means for suicide. This would argue for waiting periods.

There is evidence that men and women may respond differently to restricted access to lethal methods for suicide. A study by Leenaars and Lester (1996a) was designed, therefore, to explore whether the 1977 gun control law in Canada had different effects for men and women in their use of guns for suicide. The results indicated that the passage of C-51 seemed to have had a greater impact on women than men in the use of firearms as a method for suicide, as some men may have switched method; this phenomenon is called displacement. Men, of course, show a greater use of lethal means (WHO, 2002); firearms are often a preferred method for suicide. Suicidal women show a greater response to clinical intervention programs, educational endeavors, use of telephone crisis centers, and receiving care for psychiatric disturbances (Lester, 1995). Thus, it makes sense that this would be true with tactics of environmental control; yet research to explain the phenomenon and to developing gender-specific interventions are lacking, never mind in police.

Stack (1998), in a review of gun control studies, pointed out that gun control studies rarely take into account other societal factors (confounders) that may influence the suicide rate, such as divorce, unemployment, and the age structure of the population. A study by Leenaars, Moksony, Lester, and Wenckstern (2003) examined this critique of this public health strategy. In order to see whether social changes might have had an impact on suicide rates from guns, birth, marriage, and divorce rates as measures of domestic integration (a social variable which Durkheim,1897, argued was critical in determining suicide rates), the unemployment rate (Platt, 1984), median family income, and the percentage of the males aged 15 to 24 years as a percentage of the total male population (a group with one of Canada's highest suicide rates) were studied. The results showed that the passage of Bill C-51 in Canada in 1977, introducing stricter gun control, appeared to have been followed by a significant reduction in the suicide rate by firearms, even after controlling for the social variables. Thus, it appears that even if one controls for other social variables, gun control works.

Of course, there may have been social changes other than those considered that might be responsible for changes in the suicide rates, and the use of a different set of social indicators (such as drug use) might change the estimates of the impact of the passage of Bill C-51. However, data on such factors are not presently available. For example, alcohol and drug consumption data in Canada have only been available since 1985 (E. Simoneti, Statistics Canada, personal communication, August 19, 1999). Canada's Department of Justice (1996) has also isolated a few other social variables that may be associated with suicide in Canada, such as the percentage of foreign-born individuals and education levels, but data are not available. The role of these and other social factors should be studied in the future, if and when the necessary data become available.

Some researchers have disputed the conclusion that gun restriction has prevented suicide in Canada. Be that as it may, Carrington and Moyer (1994a, 1994b) replicated the positive findings for gun control in Ontario, and showed a similar pattern for most of Canada's provinces. All provinces had either stable or decreasing rates of firearm suicides following C-51. Results on the related phenomena of homicide (Leenaars & Lester, 2001) and accidental deaths (Leenaars & Lester, 1997b) show the same promise.

POPULATION LEVEL STUDIES: GUN CONTROL LAWS IN OTHER COUNTRIES

More research is needed to strengthen the conclusion that the passage of gun control laws in Canada, and in other countries, works. There is research, of course, elsewhere. For example, Beautrais, Fergusson, and Horwood (2006) examined the impact of more restrictive firearm legislation (Amendment to the Arms Act, 1992) in New Zealand on suicides involving firearms. The amendment restricted accessibility, required confidentiality checks of two references, and introduced more strict storage and safety requests. After the legislation, it was shown that firearm-related suicide decreased dramatically, especially in youth.

Thus, the New Zealand study not only replicated the Canadian findings, but also supported the finding that the tactic was especially useful with young people, a high-risk group for suicide globally, including in officers.

In the last 20 years or so, the positive effects of gun control laws have also been studied in the United States; these studies too support the research of Leenaars and Lester, the most comprehensive studies to date on any continent (see Lester, 2000). For example, Ludwig and Cook (2000) examined the association between guns and suicide with the implementation of the Brady Handgun Violence Protection Act. They noted a decrease of suicide by firearms in older adults (age > 55); however, there was no reduction in suicide by all methods. The authors attributed this to interim waiting periods for firearms acquisition in the Brady Law, which has since been dropped in the permanent law. Maxwell et al. (1984), Medoff and Magaddino (1983), and Sommers (1984) have also reported that restrictions in the selling and purchasing of guns played the most significant role in reduced suicide rates. These restrictions were especially important in the control of buying of guns by people with mental health disorders (psychopathology). A waiting period was also important (Medoff & Magaddino, 1983). The various studies also offered some data on the fact that these impacts were true even if one controls for some social factors. The number of factors that were studied, however, was few. This warrants caution in overgeneralizing, something Leenaars and his colleagues (2003) attempted to rectify. Thus, it is of note that waiting periods, like restriction of sale to some people, such as people with mental disorders (psychopathology) may be important. This was also noted at the individual level of analysis. One must control for psychopathology in environmental control tactics, both at an individual and societal level. Yet further studies need to explore what is effective not only at an individual level but also at national and international levels—and what about in police? (Will research ever be allowed?) The science of controlling the environment for the means is at that stage now. Probably regional differences will emerge. For example, the United States is known to be an outlier, even among developed, industrialized nations in firearm violence (Hahn et al., 2003), never mind other countries (see Hahn et al., 2003 for review of U.S. firearm laws, not only for suicide but related violent phenomena, such as homicide).

ENVIRONMENTAL CONTROL: SOME CONCLUSIONS

There are numerous studies on the impact of guns on suicide, such as firearm ownership, availability of guns, guns in the home, firearm storage, and gun control legislation (see Leenaars, 2007; Lester, 2000; Miller & Hemenway, 1999 for reviews). All these studies add to the topic of firearms and suicide. Although there have been no studies in police officers per se, studies on the availability of guns generally show that if present, the rate of use for the means of suicide increases. Ownership shows the same pattern (police have guns). Individual level studies show that the more guns in the home, the more suicides, especially in the young. Population level studies show the same patterns and associations. There are consistencies (commonalities) in the empirical studies, both individual and general. Most of the empirical studies, together with gun control law studies across the globe, show that availability of a potentially dangerous means affects the rate of use of the means for death (WHO, 2006). Firearms are a method with high case fatalities, especially in police, not only for suicide but also for homicide-suicide. The WHO (2006) identified police officers as an occupation at risk; they identified a very large environmental factor to the risk.

The tactic of controlling the environment is more complex than gun control, although it is a prototypical example. Referring to gun control as a means for suicide prevention in police in Canada and in the United States probably makes sense because it is the main method of suicide and homicide-suicide in police. It is those countries' main method of suicide. It is a highly lethal method. However, in other countries, guns are not a frequent means. Officers do not own guns in those countries. Thus, one can see great variation in means and, although gun control may make little sense in some regions of the world, the tactic of controlling the environment may well have increasing applicability, as suggested in the WHO report (Bertolote, 1993), and as studies show around the world (Leenaars et al., 2002). This is so in the United States and Canada. Firearms increase the risk of suicide and restriction of firearms decreases the risk of suicide. This would be true for at-risk officers. Thus, it follows that all police services need adequate gun control; should Lt. Michael Pigott have been able to obtain a fellow officer's gun in a locker? There can be safeguards, but also do not get lulled into the notion that no guns, no suicide. That is a fable. Our suggestions to officers: save your partner's life, control the environment.

PREVENTION: CONCLUDING REMARKS

Of greatest importance, we must understand that there are no universal formulations regarding suicide and its prevention. We can speak of understanding, but never with precision. The search for *a* singular universal response is a foolish and unrealistic fancy. There is no one implication for psychotherapy with suicidal police officers. *The* manual, *the* cookbook does not exist. (We would predict large blue walls, if a therapist used a cookbook; it is naïve—or being a "Doc Nuts" [see Danto, 1978].) The research strongly supports this opinion (Lambert, 2004; Leenaars, 2006). How do we then effectively stop the lethal suicidal officer? The answer from the research: We have to be person-centered!

One should use all measures available with highly lethal police officers; many approaches are, in fact, effective (Lambert, 2004; Leenaars, 2004). Psychotherapy can be effective with suicidal officers. This *fact* is empirically supported/validated because there are common factors that make psychotherapy effective. The seeming uniqueness of a technique is simply semantic and stylistic. The common (sameness or agreement) factors may be of overriding importance in effective psychotherapy. There are *commonalities* (Leenaars, 2006). With suicidal patients, this often implies that our treatment should also be multimodal or multicomponent. These measures may include support, cognitive-behavioral techniques, psychodynamic interpretation, medication, hospitalization, environmental control, and especially the involvement of others in the community, not only others to whom the patient was (or is) close to but also "social" agencies—the sergeant, clergy, elders, doctors, social workers, and so on—all of which serve, directly or indirectly, to alleviate the pain (American Psychiatric Association, 2003; Lambert, 2004; Leenaars, 2004; Shneidman, 1985). Suicide prevention should often be multimodal. Was the deceased officer's treatment, multimodal?

CHAPTER 8

Suicide. Homicide-Suicide. Police: Policies & Procedures

Almost 1 million people die by suicide worldwide every year; we do not know exactly how many in police, but there are many. In the United States every year, 400 police officers, at the very least, die by suicide, although it probably is twice as high. Is that true? That is far too many. Could it even be 4 times as high? In order to reduce suicide and suicidal behavior in police, many policies and procedures have been proposed and implemented. Although many of the approaches may have been/are effective, often they are not sufficiently comprehensive to address the complexity of suicide and homicide-suicide in police.

Strategies, pioneered by Gregory Zilboorg, were introduced to address this complexity in preventing suicide among police. Guidelines must be a *comprehensive and integrated approach* for the formulation and implementation of police services' strategies for prevention of suicidal behavior and the provision of supportive and rehabilitative services to officers at risk and to other affected persons, such as fellow officers and family members. *One of the hallmarks of such an approach will be collaboration* among a broad spectrum of agencies, institutions, and groups, beyond police services—and this includes a neglected group: researchers. Is that possible? How?

In the 1930s, Zilboorg had already written out such policies and procedures. A major premise for such strategies, we believe, is: Suicide cannot be isolated; it must be part of a larger mental health policy in the police service.

"No organization or government starts strategy development with a blank sheet of paper" writes Rachel Jenkins, a world leader in mental health policy, and her group (Jenkins et al., 2002). There are creative, rational, and organized ways to marshal such efforts. There are, for example, good management models of strategy development, which are critically relevant to suicide prevention in police. Police services do not need, to use a common metaphor, to reinvent the wheel. There are suggestions already available in the literature, both from police and forensic science. However, there will be key questions to ask in the establishment of policies and procedures. Here is a list of Jenkins' key questions:

http://dx.doi.org/10.2190/SHSC8

What has worked?
Can we do more of it?
What has not worked?
Can we fine tune?
Can we invest the resources elsewhere?
What elements are we uncertain about?
How do we improve evaluation so that we will know whether the various elements of the strategy are working?

The proof of the suicidological pudding is in the "ventions"—as in prevention, intervention, and postvention. In other words, the main payoff of all our efforts to prevent suicide among police lies primarily in making our policies and practice efforts more effective. That is what counts in everyday police society. This is what Rachel Jenkins, Gregory Zilboorg (already in the 1930s) and many others have called for.

We begin this chapter with a high profile media and Internet case, the suicide of Chief Thomas A. Moffatt. Once more, the unique shows what we need to do. John Carr, on that case, like a host of people—police officers, friends, family members, experts, and so on—presents some recommendations. Of course, we cannot present all, so we decided to select, verbatim, the recommendations of some main figures in the field: John Violanti, Robert Loo, and Laurence Miller. The proof of effective policies and procedures is in suicide prevention, intervention, and postvention. Violanti and Miller offer some insights on the first two, and Loo on the latter. We also suggest a must-read of the report of the International Association of Chiefs of Police (2003), *Domestic Violence by Police Officers*. Violanti also makes some of the first recommendations on homicide-suicide, borrowed from the Los Angeles Police Domestic Violence Task Force (1997).

There will be ethical issues and dilemmas, some commonly known since the 1930s (Gregory Zilboorg was, indeed, a great police suicidologist). There will be solutions, only if we have the courage and perseverance to talk about it, to break down the blue walls, and to save officers' lives. There will be challenges, but we can help Thomas, Michael, and Kelly, all suicidal officers. We first need the policies and procedures to do so, a topic that we will return to in the last chapter, wherein we present our recommendations.

* * * * * *

INTRODUCTION

On the morning of Friday, November 20, 1998, Chief Thomas A. Moffatt of the Central Falls, Rhode Island, Police Department, drove his police vehicle to police headquarters. He waved to passing police officers (dissembling). He drove to his assigned spot in a garage. Several minutes later, two officers walking past the vehicle noticed the chief in his car. They greeted him; however, Chief Moffatt did not return the greeting. They approached the vehicle, to find the chief slumped in the seat. His service pistol was on the seat. Unable to enter, they contacted the fire department. Subsequently, Chief Moffatt was pronounced dead by apparent gun shot wound. The death was later determined to be a suicide (Carr, 2001).

The senior officer, Commander Rudolph Leganza, was called to the "crime scene," and subsequently joined by Mayor Lee Matthews. Understandably, with both police and fire department personnel traumatized, Commander Leganza was left with the difficult task of informing everyone; he notified the chief's family and other service personnel before media disclosure. The Commander and Mayor drove to the Moffatt home and met/informed his wife and daughter, who is a police officer. The aftershocks, the skeletons grew (Carr, 2001).

Ongoing investigation, including by the media, prolonged the posttraumatic reactions. The pain of Chief Moffatt became the pain of the survivors. The question of "why?" was figural, a most typical reaction after such events. It was learned that the chief had a gambling addiction. "Unable or unwilling to seek assistance," his addiction affected his personal and professional life. He dissembled. He borrowed money; he misappropriated funds. On the morning of his suicide, a meeting with state union officials and Chief Moffatt was to take place. Ethical issues arose. There was probably disgrace, maybe even anxiety and depression. He had had an untarnished 30-year career in policing. He must have felt disgraced. He wanted to escape (Carr, 2001). Did the blue walls prevent him from getting help? Since the 1930s, there have been common facts: blue walls are killing officers. Why do officers not express their pain? Why do they kill themselves? Or kill others, followed by self? Police express less and are more guarded; they are more indirect. They do everyday. Is it expected in the blue culture? Why is dissembling *the* most common observation, for some 80 years plus? Can interventions be undertaken? What have we learned about the lethal stimuli implications of indirect expressions?

The fact that police may express more indirectness may be expected from research to date across cultures (Leenaars, 2008) and also from a broader blue culture. Some cultures do dissemble more. Police collective culture encourages police, and thus suicidal police officers, to adhere to the macho tradition, including in matters of suicide. There is great stigmatization regarding self-harm and psychopathology in police. People, in fact, take pride in the blue collective style, but maybe for suicidal people, it fosters not communicating pain and suicidal intent, not even being conscious of individual pain. The indirectness may, thus, add to the lethal mix in a vulnerable and self-harsh officer. It may well be that police beliefs foster indirectness of expressing intrapsychic pain, emotional disturbance, and so on. Individualism is not fostered in the culture, blue relatedness is. The suicidal state may, thus, be more veiled, clouded, or guarded. This is what we have called dissembling or masking and is, we believe, a significant factor in police suicide risk and police homicide-suicide risk. In police, we believe, there are more unconscious dynamics, even self-deception; there are more reasons for the suicide than the officer expresses and is maybe consciously aware of. Further, based on research since the 1930s, we can speculate that these dynamics in officers may be associated to collectivistic blue processes of being a police officer, but this speculation is only provisional. Yet Zilboorg, Danto, Violanti, Loo, and many others have stated so; we agree. Research is needed, but will it be allowed? Why does administration allow officers to kill themselves? Why, since the 1930s, have they done little?

At times there have been constructive actions. Carr (2001), who reported the Chief Moffatt case, noted that intervention was undertaken. The suicide of that chief executive officer was the impetus for intervention. Survivors were assisted, a necessity after such an event (Carr, 2001). Postvention was implemented; a must.

The best intervention is prevention, a basic, as presented early in suicidology, at the very beginning of the science (Shneidman & Farberow, 1957). As Carr (2001) noted, the suicide of Thomas Moffatt had implications; so does the suicide or homicide-suicide of officers. Police services can prevent many such needless deaths. Zilboorg stated so in 1940!

The very aim of psychological investigations, retrospective or otherwise, into police suicide is to turn the tragedy into something positive. This is the request of every survivor. Many people, not just survivors, hope to do so. We can do so in different ways: here, we present in this review some highlights from the available literature. Does it help to understand? Once we know what suicide is and what homicide-suicide is, we can make better recommendations to prevent a future tragedy, a suicide or a suicide following homicide in police. Our aim, like all prevention efforts in this field, is to prevent further human misery.

POLICIES AND PROCEDURES FOR PREVENTION AND INTERVENTION

Understandably, there has been a host of people, including police officers, friends, family members, and so on, who have presented some recommendations for prevention. Everyone wants to prevent an *Othello* event. Of course, we cannot present all, so we decided to select, verbatim, the recommendations of three major figures in the field: John Violanti (2001, 2007), Robert Loo (2001), and Laurence Miller (2005). We conclude with some thoughts by Dennis Conroy (2001) on developing a plan. Finally, our plan would also include the recommendations from the report of the International Association of Chiefs of Police (2003), *Domestic Violence by Police Officers*. Every officer should read that complete report. We hope that these ideas will guide the necessary healing.

Violanti (2001) recommended the following:

SUICIDE PREVENTION ISSUES

A Police Suicide Prevention Model

Because suicide is likely to the result of a complex interaction of many factors, all major components of the work environment must necessarily be involved in its prevention. Loo (1986) and Silverman and Felner (1995) comment that a suicide prevention approach should focus on suicide, as well as building a person's work and life competencies, thereby enhancing their resilience to stressors. The following is a proposal for a suicide prevention model:

Psychological Assessment

Although recruit screening in most major police departments involves psychological testing, quite often other personal and social factors are not considered. Loo (1995), for example, stated that predisposing personality factors or precipitating family history (family violence, substance abuse) should be noted for tracking high-risk officers in the future.

Tracking High-Risk Officers

Loo (1995) has suggested that police departments develop criteria to identify and track high-risk officers (such as officers with marital difficulties, substance abuse, work problems and other life problems) so that timely support can be provided prior to suicide. A behavioral profile based on these indicators should be established for each officer and should be reviewed every 6 months to determine which officers are possibly at risk for suicide.

Access to Firearms

Certainly, the risk of suicide increases in police officers because they have access to firearms. This author's data revealed that 95% of police suicides were by firearm (Violanti et al., 1996). The practice of some departments of requiring police to carry firearms off duty may be an important target for police organizational policy change because such immediate access can facilitate impulsive suicidal tendencies in high-risk officers.

Family Involvement

Seminars should be given to police recruits and their families so they understand the effects of police work. Ivanoff (1994), for example, found that 58% of police suicides in New York City were the result of relationship problems with family or significant others. Counseling services should be made available to families and officers.

Training

Training can help officers and avoid psychological factors leading to suicide. Ivanoff (1994) suggested that police suicide training programs include recognition of psychological depression, communication skills, conflict resolution and intimate-relationship maintenance.

> **Stress Awareness**
>
> Stress awareness is a psychologically sound method to help individuals cope with stress. A well-rounded stress-education program should include identification of stress, the value and techniques of physical exercise, benefits of proper nutrition, interpersonal communication methods and coping styles.
>
> **Professional Intervention**
>
> Not only can an effective intervention effort save police officers' lives, but it also can safeguard agencies from the devastating effects of suicide. To help officers take the first difficult step to intervention, the police organization should develop and increase accessibility to confidential psychological services. Essentially, officers need a safe place out of administrative view to go for help. It is necessary to establish a professional network of psychologists or psychiatrists who are familiar with police problems. When troubled members are in need of such services, they can be referred easily.
>
> **Retirement Counseling**
>
> Retirement is not an easy transition for most people and it is even more difficult for police officers. Gaska (1980) calculated a 10-fold risk of suicide among Detroit police retirees over the general population. The cohesiveness of police officers and the "protection" that being part of the police culture provides are lost upon separation from police service. (Violanti, 1992; Violanti, 2001, pp. 442–444)

Miller (2005), in his review on the topic (see also Mohandie & Hatcher, 1999), suggested the following:

> **Preventing Police Suicide**
>
> Invoking the principle that "the best form of crisis intervention is crisis prevention" (Miller, 1998; Miller, 2006b), law enforcement agencies can do much in the initial stages of selecting and acculturating their officers to mitigate the predisposing factors for officer stress, depression, and suicide (Baker & Baker, 1996; Mohandie & Hatcher, 1999; Mohandie et al., 1996; Zelig, 1996).
>
> Psychological screening is an important part of the selection process for new officers to ensure that these officers possess a reasonable degree of psychological stability and maturity. Periodic reassessments should also be part of the personnel standard operating procedure to assure that budding problems don't sprout unobserved into major crises. This also presupposes an efficient, nonstigmatized referral system for dealing with officers in psychological distress, so that any problems observed can receive appropriate treatment in a supportive atmosphere. One way of reducing stigmatization and encouraging troubled officers to come forward for help is via education about police stress, depression, and suicide, provided by means of inservice programs or outside continuing education.
>
> Finally, healthy law enforcement organizations contribute to the overall psychological health and resilience of their officers by reinforcing fair practices and open communication among levels of the organization (Peak et al.,

2004; Thibault et al., 2004). This applies to virtually all public and private organizations, not just law enforcement agencies (Miller, 1998; Miller, in press, pp. 103–104).

Violanti (2007), specifically on homicide-suicide, borrowing from the Los Angeles Police Domestic Violence Task Force (1997), recommended the following:

- Create specialized unit within Internal Affairs Division with the primary responsibility of conducting investigations of officers involved in domestic violence situations.
- Treat offending police officers no differently than any other citizen. A crime report should be taken in every instance where a crime is alleged or there exists evidence that a crime occurred. Make an arrest in every legally mandated instance.
- Refer every domestic violence investigation with prima facie evidence of criminal misconduct to the appropriate prosecuting agency in a timely manner.
- Do not discontinue domestic violence investigations merely because the victim recants or indicates unwillingness to testify in disciplinary hearings.
- Mandate termination of employees in serious cases of domestic violence where officers demonstrate by a convincing pattern that they cannot control their abusive conduct.
- Increase suspensions for sustained acts of domestic violence in length and severity. Mete out long-term suspensions or terminations to those who have repeated instances of sustained allegations.
- Document sustained allegations of misconduct and consider them in performance reviews and promotions.
- Develop a Batterers Program under the direction of the Behavioral Science Services Section. Require contracts to include mandatory counseling in all sustained complaints involving domestic violence. (pp. 102–103)

POLICIES AND PROCEDURES FOR POSTVENTION

Loo (2001), focusing on postvention, recommended the following:

Effective Postvention for Police Suicide:

Shneidman (1981b) coined the term postvention, in contrast to prevention, to describe the sorts of actions taken after a suicide largely to help survivors such as family, friends, and coworkers. Postvention was seen as a natural extension to the established suicide prevention field partly because there will always be some base level of suicide even when highly effective suicide prevention programs exist and partly because the survivors of suicide can be viewed as victims of post-traumatic stress (i.e., post traumatic stress disorder: PTSD) and, therefore, in need of assistance in dealing with their grief reaction.

Survivor Reactions to Police Suicide

The signs and symptoms of distress and bereavement resulting from the suicide of an officer might be a mix of any of the following commonly-reported reactions among survivors (American Psychiatric Association, 1994):

- shock over the suicide;
- feelings of grief;
- feelings of helplessness;
- feelings of abandonment, isolation, and loneliness;
- feelings of depression and weepiness;
- feelings of guilt because they believe that they might have been able to prevent the suicide;
- sexual dysfunction;
- suicidal thoughts . . . the contagion effect
- anger toward the suicided, the police department, other survivors, or the media;
- a loss of interest in work, family and friends, and other activities;
- increased work absences; lateness, and use of sick leave;
- alcohol and drug abuse; and
- disruptive sleep and eating patterns.

Steps in Suicide Postvention

The major steps in postvention should include any or all of the following depending upon the circumstances.

- Establish and execute your standard operating procedure (SOP) for postvention. The SOP should specify the key positions/persons responsible for initiating the SOP. For example, the immediate supervisor, the officer who first hears about the suicide (e.g., the duty officer), the departmental psychologist/health professional, padre/clergy, and internal affairs.
- Have a crisis team trained and ready to have a planning meeting to initiate the Critical Incident Stress Debriefing (CISD). The team could be a mix of health professionals and trained peer counselors.
- Notify the departmental administration, next-of-kin, family physician and clergy if known, and other key persons.
- A departmental communication release should be made as soon as practical to let fellow officers and staff know the facts rather than have the grapevine circulate rumors. Manage the external media by having a timely press release so that facts rather than rumors reach the media.
- Have a carefully picked debriefing facility readily available. While it may be practical to use a room in a police facility, an off-site facility such as a meeting or conference room in a community center, might be better for the survivors.
- Do at least one follow-up session to address unresolved concerns and any new issues that arose since the debriefing.
- Conduct a confidential evaluation of the postvention by having participants complete, for example, a confidential and anonymous evaluation questionnaire a week or two after the debriefing to identify particularly what worked

well and what needs to be improved for future postventions. Alternatively, the evaluation might be conducted as a group session thus allowing for interactions among survivors but precluding anonymity.

Ethical Issues and Dilemmas

The issue of suicide contagion is important because police are armed and can readily commit suicide in an impulsive but undo-able moment. Police supervisors and health professionals must be alert to any warning signs (e.g., verbalizations about committing suicide, mood changes such as becoming despondent) that a survivor himself/herself is experiencing suicidal ideation or intent. Such persons must be referred to a qualified health professional in suicide prevention (unnumbered).

Of course, as in any service, evaluation of prevention, intervention, and postvention services will play an integral part (Loo, 2001; Miller, 2005; Violanti, 2001, 2007). Our efforts need to be empirically based. This book is only one step; there is a lot of work to do. Police services need to *persevere*, a hallmark of wellness.

CONCLUDING REMARKS

Finally, police services need to develop a plan of action with clear goals and objectives; they need to develop a protocol for dealing with police suicide and police suicide-homicide (Conroy, 2001). This appears to be especially true when services have gone through the suicide of, say, Lt. Michael Pigott or a homicide followed by the suicide of an officer, such as in the case of, say, David Lucio and Kelly Johnson. We hope the thoughts from the general literature will help us not only to understand the following challenge, "We ought to know what we are preventing," but also the challenge, "We have to know who you are helping." These are great challenges. We hope that we have brought the reader, whether an officer or not, a little closer to that plan. Regardless of what the policies and procedures will be, they have to be grounded in evidence-based study (Brent, 1989; Leenaars, 2004; Seltzer et al., 2001; Shneidman, 1977). Ultimately, we believe that suicide and homicide-suicide can be prevented. As already seen in the 1930s in New York, our greatest obstacle will be the many blue walls. We need to get past the stigma of suicide, homicide-suicide, emotional disturbance, and some specifically blue stigmas, but so does the world. Police have to own the problem, otherwise nothing will get done. We cannot wait for some Chief, some Police Board, Interpol, the FBI, the RCMP, and so on. We, police and those of us who are not police, but working with them on multidisciplinary teams for forensic investigations; providing mental health services to the officers and their families; administrating to such officers; surviving a suicide or homicide-suicide in police officers; providing survivor/bereavement services after the death by suicide (which includes homicide-suicide); and many more, need to own the problem; nothing will get done otherwise. Suicide among police has, and can be, prevented. The police officer does not have to die.

CHAPTER 9

Suicide. Homicide-Suicide. Police: A Public Case

Following Shneidman, we present this case, *res ipsa loquitur*. Let the public report speak for itself.

* * * * * *

Report to the
London Police Service and
London Community on the Deaths of
David Lucio and Kelly Johnson

Authors:

Antoon A. Leenaars, Ph.D., C. Psych., CPQ
Windsor, Ontario

Peter Collins, M.C.A., M.D., F.R.C.P.©)
Ontario Provincial Police & University of Toronto

Deborah Sinclair, MSW, RSW
Toronto, Ontario

Prepared for:
Chief Murray Faulkner
London Police Service

May 20, 2008

http://dx.doi.org/10.2190/SHSC9

OVERVIEW OF COMMITTEE MANDATE

Opening Statement: *The committee wishes to express sincere condolences to the family and friends of David Lucio, to the family and friends of Kelly Johnson, and to the police officers and staff of the London Police Service. We also thank them for their cooperation, not only to understand the tragic events, but also for their input into the recommendations. We also recognize the profound effect that the tragedy has had on the London community.*

David Lucio died by homicide on the June 7th, 2007. Kelly Johnson died by suicide following the homicide of David Lucio on the June 7th, 2007. They had been police officers of the London Police Service. Chief Murray Faulkner, LPS, on June 11th, 2007, released the following report to the public:

> "As a result of a case conference and extensive investigation involving members of the Regional Coroners Office, the Pathologist and the London Police Service, the Coroner has determined that retired Superintendent David Lucio died as a result of sustaining a single gunshot wound. The investigative findings indicate that the passenger of the vehicle, Acting Inspector Kelly Johnson, fired the gunshot that killed David Lucio prior to taking her own life with a single gunshot. As a result this tragic incident has been determined to be a murder/suicide."

The London Police Service, as part of its response, established a committee, with Dr. Antoon A. Leenaars, Dr. Peter Collins, and Ms. Deborah Sinclair, to investigate and examine this tragic murder/suicide. The background of the committee members is summarized in Appendix A of this report. On July 9th, 2007, Chief Murray Faulkner requested an examination of the following:

- "The extent to which the murder/suicide was predictable and preventable.
- What safeguards could be in place to reduce the risk of future incidents?"

A psychological autopsy was conducted as part of this review. A psychological autopsy involves an analysis of available data and evidence, such as personal documents, reports, electronic mail, and third-party interviews to understand the reasons and dynamics underlying a tragedy. In this matter the psychological autopsy was developed in the context of David Lucio's and Kelly Johnson's lives and addressed the fundamental questions, 'Why did the homicide-suicide happen?' and 'What can we do to prevent a similar occurrence?'

Throughout our investigation, the committee has taken its responsibilities very seriously and acted diligently with the charge of not only understanding the tragedy but also for making recommendations that will hopefully save lives in the future with regard to suicide and homicide-suicide at the London Police Service or other police services who may face similar circumstances.

Homicide-suicide is a complex and multi-determined event. People are naturally perplexed, stressed, confused and overwhelmed when they are confronted by a homicide-suicide. These thoughts and feelings are especially true in the tragic David Lucio/Kelly Johnson homicide-suicide, both well-known and respected senior police officers. Understandably, homicide-suicide, given its complexity, is most difficult to understand. It is a rare event and even more rare to have the perpetrator a woman. There is in fact, only one study on female perpetrators of homicide-suicide. In a recent US study, 95% of the perpetrators in a homicide-suicide were men who acted most often in the context of family and intimate relationships.

There were a number of contributing factors in the Lucio/Johnson homicide-suicide: emotional disturbance, historical stressors (diagnosis of her mother's illness), stress (the loss/rejection of David Lucio that probably resulted in unbearable distress and anxiety), alcohol abuse, and the availability of a firearm. There are common aspects of homicide-suicide, such as domestic violence, that were not evident in this case. There was no evidence of domestic violence between David Lucio and Kelly Johnson.

Kelly Johnson was unable to adjust to her life's demands. At the time before her death, she was "desperate." She had not been eating or sleeping, was experiencing "panics," was drinking alcohol often, was depressed and was not coping well. She appears to have had both generalized anxiety and separation anxiety. She was observed to be depressed and "emotional" at times, but also masked or hid her emotions, thoughts and intentions. Kelly Johnson was observed to be a capable friend and employee and there were no clues to suicide or homicide-suicide. No professional involved with Kelly Johnson, her friends, family or colleagues had any foresight of the lethal circumstances and impending tragedy.

A main conclusion is that at the time of her death, Kelly Johnson possessed the characteristics and dynamics more like a person who died by suicide than a female perpetrator of homicide. Kelly Johnson's death was a suicide; one must adopt that point of view to understand her. She had the following intrapsychic characteristics of suicide: unbearable psychological pain, cognitive constriction (or narrow thinking), indirect expressions (or ambivalence), emotional disturbance, and a feeling of being vulnerable. She had the following interpersonal characteristics: problematic relationships, rejection-aggression and the wish to escape. In too many Canadians, suicide becomes the only solution, and in a very small group, homicide-suicide becomes the best solution. These terms are defined in Appendix B of this report. She also had some of the markers for intimate partner homicide-suicide, such as frustrated personal relationships, ambivalence, jealousy, separation, depression, helplessness, and guilt. However many aspects of Kelly Johnson and these circumstances were rare and unique and made any prediction difficult. Suicide among police, in Canada, occurs but is less than in the general population. The incidences of suicide in policing is higher in other countries.

Although there is little research on homicide-suicide, among police there appears to have a higher occurrence than in the general population. We hope our report and recommendations are a step toward a better understanding of these complex issues.

EXECUTIVE SUMMARY

During the summer of 2004 David Lucio and Kelly Johnson were both married to their long-term spouses. It was during this summer that Kelly Johnson's mother was diagnosed with cancer. This diagnosis was devastating for Kelly Johnson as she and her mother were very close. Shortly after this diagnosis Kelly Johnson and David Lucio began an intimate extramarital relationship. This relationship continued until June 2007 and led to the dissolution of both marriages. During this time a number of other significant events occurred, which had a traumatic effect on Kelly Johnson. In December of 2005 Kelly Johnson's mother succumbed to her illness and passed away. Her pet of fifteen years also passed away, and she also dealt with on-going relationship issues as she and David Lucio parted ways so that she could attempt reconciliation with her husband. This attempt was short lived as David Lucio and Kelly Johnson continued their relationship during this reconciliation.

During this time Kelly Johnson had sought professional counseling, first through the London Employee Assistance Consortium, and then with a private counselor. In the weeks preceding June 7th, 2007 a number of things occurred to create additional stress for her. Kelly Johnson's ex-husband was retiring from his position as Inspector of the Professional Standards Branch, which meant Kelly Johnson would no longer have ready access to him at work. To complicate matters Kelly Johnson was being promoted to the rank of Inspector and was taking over for her ex-husband in Professional Standards as his retirement facilitated her promotion.

At the same time David Lucio's daughter, who worked outside the country, was in London for two weeks. David Lucio and his estranged wife spent time with their daughter as a family, which meant David Lucio was less available to Kelly Johnson. The Lucio's re-connected during this time and decided to give their marriage another chance. David Lucio told friends that he was ending his relationship with Kelly Johnson after his daughter left to return to work. There is no doubt that the relationship between David Lucio and Kelly Johnson ended on Monday June 4th, although some may argue about who ended the relationship. It is clear that on June 5th and 6th Kelly Johnson was in a very fragile state. She was highly perturbed and was not eating or sleeping. Close friends were concerned about her. Upon analysis after the tragedy, her electronic mail reflected emotionality, narrow thinking and other indicators of suicidal ideation.

On June 6th Kelly Johnson went to David Lucio's residence for the evening and sent an electronic mail to David Lucio from his own computer (David Lucio was not at his residence when the electronic mail was sent). The electronic mail was very desperate in nature, requesting that David Lucio and Kelly Johnson reconcile under whatever terms David Lucio would find acceptable. This electronic mail was opened by David Lucio at 9:50 P.M. and no one knows what occurred between this time and just prior to midnight when Kelly Johnson had David Lucio drive her to the London Police Service Headquarters where she retrieved her service pistol and subsequently shot David Lucio and then herself.

The Independent Review Committee is of the view that these deaths were neither predictable nor preventable by the London Police Service or other individuals associated with David Lucio and Kelly Johnson. These findings are based on the following facts.

1. Kelly Johnson was seen by a mental health professional just prior to the tragedy and that professional did not document Kelly Johnson to be at risk for suicide or homicide. Although she attended appointments, with professionals, overall it appears that she was non-compliant with treatment. The non-compliance reference is in relation to the fact that she was attending counseling but perhaps not discussing the depth of her problems, as well as, being prescribed medication, but concerned about the side effects and did not follow through with the prescribed treatment.
2. Kelly Johnson had been seen by her family doctor, who diagnosed her as having an adjustment disorder relating to her mother's illness. She was also perceived to be depressed but was not viewed as being a threat to herself or others. She was also seen by the London Police Service employee assistance plan, London Employee Assistance Consortium counsellor who did not deem her a risk to herself or others in prior years.
3. David Lucio was a highly skilled retired senior police officer and apparently did not suspect anything on June 7th, 2007, in spite of the recent relationship break up. He was aware of Kelly Johnson's distress about the break up. He also spent the evening with her and drove her to the police station enroute to her residence. Clearly he did not suspect that she would be picking up her service pistol.
4. Kelly Johnson received ongoing positive evaluations from supervisors and peers and had just been promoted to Acting Inspector of the Professional Standards Branch. There were no warning signs in the workplace of a pending tragedy.

Although this tragedy was neither predictable nor preventable in our opinion, there are a number of issues that Kelly Johnson was dealing with which have only come to light with the benefit of hindsight and access to critical information from professionals, friends, family, colleagues, and most importantly, information gleaned from the psychological autopsy. The psychological autopsy that reviewed all the information after the tragedy concluded she was suicidal. These issues were identified and followed by recommendations, which flow from the facts of this tragedy.

RECOMMENDATIONS

These recommendations flow from the findings of the Review Committee. The recommendations are based on the facts as we understand them. One of the major reflections in our review is in the area of mental health and the stigma surrounding mental health, which in many cases leads to barriers to seeking help. Police officers are no different from society at large in facing problems in regards to mental health. Police are not exempt from being perpetrators and potential victims of domestic violence. The Review Committee believes that prevention is the best intervention and education is the best tool to achieve this outcome. The Review Committee supports education and initiatives through training opportunities, which would reduce barriers to seeking help.

1. The London Police Service should continue to be committed to the mental health and well being of all its members. The London Police Service could explore an expansion of services by innovative models such as the Psychological Services Section in some larger police services (e.g. Calgary Police Service). The mandate of this section could include being a support to members experiencing emotional difficulties through early intervention. The London Police Service could consider hiring a Police Psychologist to manage the section. We recommend that a committee be established to determine the framework for such a section, realizing that the London Police Service may not have the need for a full time psychologist or the resources to fund a full time section based on the model of larger police services.
2. The London Police Service should continue to build liaisons with the London Employee Assistance Consortium and other community services, to help prevent, intervene and address aftermaths of suicide and other traumatic events.
3. The London Police Service should continue to support ready access to psychological, medical and empirically based interventions. Furthermore, the London Police Service should prepare a list of senior counselors in the community with experience in dealing with police officers. This list should be re-compiled on an on-going basis and be readily available to officers to compliment the existing employee assistance plan.
4. On the recommendation of the committee, the London Police Service has already implemented a more comprehensive psychological assessment for recruiting, the Minnesota Multiphasic Personality Inventory-2 (MMPI-2), with inclusion of the revised clinical scales. The latter scales are most effective in screening a wide array of risks. Furthermore, the committee

recommends that additional re-assessment be undertaken at the promotional level and when members are transferred to higher stress areas such as Emergency Response Section, Drug Units, Cyber Crime Units, Forensic Identification and fatal motor vehicle collision investigations.

5. The committee recognizes the London Police Service document, "Handling of Firearms"; it clearly articulates the safe storage, discharge, handling and transportation of firearms. Kelly Johnson's behaviour was a clear violation of this procedure. We do not advocate further gun controls measures. We recommend that London Police Service continue to remove access to firearms for officers who are off duty due to a stress related illness or mental disturbance. Policies should be developed to determine if and when officers should have access to firearms upon their return to work.

   Notwithstanding our review, it is important to note another police officer homicide-suicide in Eastern Ontario in 2004. Upon review, the Chief Coroner suggested supervised control of issue firearms when officers are off duty. While police services have not found this policy change to be a feasible and practical solution to date, the Lucio-Johnson tragedy affords the London Police Service and other police services the opportunity to re-examine this issue. The costs and practical implications of such a new policy may make this recommendation difficult to implement but we feel that a study together with other organizations such as the Ontario Association of Chiefs of Police may be helpful to thoroughly address the issue. As with all policies regarding weapons, it is necessary to weigh the practical, physical, and financial implications of undertaking changes for such a large police service against the obvious likelihood that supervised control might have altered the outcome of this particular tragedy.

6. The London Police Service should develop a clear policy on conflict of interest; regulations and procedures need to be developed and implemented. We recommend that the London Police Service develop a committee to establish such regulations and procedures including a clear personnel policy regarding conflict of interest involving related members. These should not restrict officers' rights, but also London Police Service's policies need to eliminate any actual or potential conflict of interest in the workplace, which may arise from a working relationship between immediate family members and/or intimate partners.

7. The London Police Service should develop new initiatives to deal with vicarious trauma and stress management for police personnel. There needs to be greater awareness and recognition to the unique demands facing female police officers in a male dominated police profession.

8. Postvention refers to those interventions after the tragic event has occurred and deals with the traumatic after-effects. In this case, these effects refer not only to family, friends and fellow officers, but the entire London community. We recommend that the London Police Service, together with

community experts, develop comprehensive efforts for postvention in response to this tragedy.

9. We recommend that for those individuals who would like to gain a better understanding of suicide, and homicide-suicide review the selected readings that were used to form the basis of this report be made available to any person who wishes to review them. These could be kept in hardcopy form in the London Police Service library and made accessible via an Internet link. We believe that it is important to ensure ongoing education for all police personnel and their families on domestic violence, suicide, mental health issues, substance abuse, health and wellness and the aspects unique to police culture including strengths and stressors. The following website is recommended: http://www.suicideinfo.ca
   Request topic: homicide-suicide

APPENDIX A: Committee Authors

Antoon A. Leenaars, Ph.D., C.Psych.

Dr. Antoon A. Leenaars is a psychologist in private practice in mental health and public health, Windsor. He is the first Past President of the Canadian Association for Suicide Prevention (CASP), and a Past President of the American Association of Suicidology (AAS). He has published 11 books, including, *Psychotherapy with Suicidal People* (2004), and was the founding/first Editor-in-Chief of *Archives of Suicide Research,* the official journal of the International Academy for Suicide Research (IASR). He has consulted for the World Health Organization (WHO), and has provided forensic services on cases of wrongful death, suicide, homicide, and homicide-suicide for police services and legal institutions.

Peter Collins, MCA, MD, FRCP©)

Dr Collins is the forensic psychiatrist with the Ontario Provincial Police and a staff forensic psychiatrist with the Law and Mental Health Program at the Centre of Addiction and Mental Health in Toronto. Dr. Collins obtained his Masters in Applied Criminology from the University of Ottawa, his Medical Degree from McMaster University and completed his postgraduate medical training in Psychiatry at the University of Toronto. He is an Associate Professor with the Department of Psychiatry, Faculty of Medicine at the University of Toronto. He is an expert on violent crime and has lectured, and worked with, criminal justice agencies internationally, including the FBI, the U.S. Department of Homeland Security, Interpol and Europol.

Deborah Sinclair, MSW, RSW

Ms. Sinclair is a social worker with an independent practice in Toronto. She has been involved in clinical work and training in the area of domestic violence for over 30 years. She has provided workshops on violence, trauma and vicarious trauma across Canada and the US. Ms. Sinclair has been involved in writing and developing education programs for police, child protection workers and crisis workers across the country. She is a founding member of the Ontario Chief Coroner's Domestic Violence Death Review Committee, which is the only committee of its kind in Canada.

APPENDIX B:
Glossary of Terms

Access to Firearms:
Access to firearms greatly increases the lethality in suicidal persons.

Cognitive Constriction (or Narrow Thinking):
Tunnel vision, or rigid thinking, is common and one of the deadliest aspects of the suicidal state. The individual sees suicide as the one and only solution for their current difficulties. They think everything is hopeless and things will never be better.

Domestic Violence:
Refers to any behaviour within an intimate relationship that causes physical, psychological, or sexual harm to those in the relationship

Emotional Disturbance (or Psychopathology):
About 60-90% of suicidal people have a psychiatric disorder, the most common being depression or psychosis.

Indirect expression (or Ambivalence):
The suicidal person is deeply ambivalent about living or dying.

Interpersonal Relations (Problem Relationships):
The suicidal person often feels alone and cut off from others. They have experienced conflict and rejection from others.

Intrapsychic:
Existing or taking place within the mind or psyche.

Rejection/Aggression:
An experience of loss or rejection (for example, spouse leaving, fired from job, ill health, death of a fellow officer) is often a trigger for suicide. Research suggests that those who react with anger or aggression may be more at risk for suicide. Suicide is an act of self-directed violence; homicide-suicide is an act of other-directed violence and self-directed violence.

Unbearable psychological pain:
The common trigger for suicide is unbearable pain, a deep anguish, in which the person feels hopeless and helpless.

CHAPTER 10

Recommendations for the Prevention/Intervention/Postvention of Suicide. Homicide-Suicide. Police

The classical approach to *prevention*, whether mental health or public health, as we have learned, is prevention/intervention/postvention:

Prevention. Prevention is education. Research shows that educating police officers, professionals, and the general public about the fact that suicide is a problem, that there is a stigma, what clues to look for, and where to get help, is effective.

Intervention. Intervention is the care and treatment of the officer who is in crisis or who has a suicidal intent. Officers can help; nonetheless, professionally trained people—psychologists, psychiatrists, GPs, social workers, crisis workers, nurses, and so on—continue to play the primary roles in intervention, and the psychologists/psychiatrists with police services belonging on this list. *Psychotherapy*, medication, hospitalization, and controlling the environment (such as gun control) have been shown to be a very important part of the supportive treatments for those at risk. Despite our attempt to present some common recommendations on intervention, any effort has to have local direction to be effective. It takes a police service and community. There is a lot that needs to be done with police officers, especially addressing the stigma and the blue walls.

Postvention. Postvention is what we do after someone has died by suicide. Suicide can profoundly affect family, friends, and fellow officers. There can be feelings of guilt, shock, anger, and *even contagion suicide* (this is high in police). There is such a sting. Police psychologists, along with others trained in this type of care, can provide therapeutic support for those who have lost a loved one to suicide. The pain can be mollified.

* * * * * *

INTRODUCTION

We wish to acknowledge the writings of the following people, Nancy Allen (1980), John Violanti (2001, 2007), and Robert Loo (2001) in the recommendations; we borrow here and there from their work on the topic. Much of our

http://dx.doi.org/10.2190/SHSC10

recommendations are common in police services. There are commonalities. We also wish to thank Dr. Peter Collins, Ontario Provincial Police, and Dr. Adriana Celser, Calgary Police Service; their help was extensive to the recommendations.

We hereby offer our recommendations in prevention, intervention, and postvention.

PREVENTION

I Despite police and community efforts, we believe that more needs to be done to prevent future events. Prevention consists of strategies to ameliorate the conditions that lead to suicide and homicide-suicide (Shneidman, 1973). This is primarily education, but not only. The best intervention is prevention, a basic in the field. Such education is enormously complex and from the ecological view, involves mental health promotion beyond the police services. Based on our findings, the area can be reasonably divided into the following: Mental Health: General; Prevention, Training, Liaison and Programs; Alcohol/ Drug Abuse; Professional and Ethical Challenges (such as the specific challenge of blue walls).

Mental Health: General

1. Not only the local police services, but also the national and international police services, should support efforts that result in breaking down barriers/walls to suicide prevention, such as blue walls. This should include addressing issues of stigma regarding mental health condition/ emotional disturbances/stress, suicidality, and help-seeking that are common barriers and blue barriers to wellness (Canada's Standing Committee on Social Affairs, Services & Technology, 2006; Department of Health, U.K., 2002; Jenkins et al., 2002; Satcher, 1998; U.S. Department of Health and Human Services, 2001).
2. Police services should be committed to ensuring the mental health and well being of all its members and their families, and accomplish this by providing psychological assessments, counselling and therapy, facilitated by an established or to-be-established Psychological Services Section. We recommend the following:
   - Included in the mandate of the Psychological Services Section is the prevention or lessening of the potential negative psychological impact of a diagnosed mental health condition on the member and his or her family; and the prevention, lessening, managing and addressing the risk that may be associated with a diagnosed emotional disturbance (psychopathology).
   - Police services should encourage early intervention for members experiencing emotional difficulties so that support can be provided at

the earliest possible time, including assessment, psychotherapy, and, as needed, support through appropriate psychopharmacological treatment, environmental control, and hospitalization.

- Although most police services have peer support programs, these become mandatory in suicide prevention. Fellow officers, after psychological assessment (see Assessment below), should be trained in suicide *prevention* and mental health in general, within the Psychological Services Section. Peer programs should be integrated in the following policies and procedures. (Don't underestimate fellow officers in preventing suicide!)
- Members discharged from a psychiatric or health facility will contact the Psychological Services Section.

To achieve this, we suggest that services that have not done so, develop a committee to establish/review such a service. This will include issues of definition, general, creation of patient relationship, peer programs, and confidentiality. We here offer a definition:

Definition

- A diagnosed mental health condition (psychopathology) is a condition that meets the definition criteria in the Diagnostic and Statistical Manual of Mental Disorders.

3. First and foremost, not only for prevention, but also intervention and postvention, a police service, if not already done, should hire a police Psychologist (under the model that the police service chooses to establish), following the recommendations of such since the beginning of study on police suicide. This is consistent with recommendation #2, which we will further address here and there below. It is paramount that the individual with a PhD or equivalent is experienced (minimum 5 years) in psychology and forensics/policing.

Prevention, Training, Liaison, and Programs

4. The police service should train all police officers in suicide and its prevention. The suicide training program should include recognition of emotional disturbances, police stress, posttraumatic reactions, suicide clues, and prevention strategies. The individual's work and life competencies should be fostered, thereby enhancing officers' resilience to stress.
5. The police service should continue to build liaison(s) with community services, to help prevent, intervene, and address aftermaths of suicide and other traumatic events.

6. Police services should train police officers in the prevention of domestic violence (see International Association of Chiefs of Police [2003] document, a policy of the IACP response to violence in women project).
7. Although most police services have addressed domestic violence, we support the following suggestions of Violanti (2007), specifically for homicide-suicide. Violanti recommended:
   - Create a specialized unit within Internal Affairs Division with the primary responsibility of conducting investigations of officers involved in domestic violence situations.
   - Treat offending police officers no differently than any other citizen. A crime report should be taken in every instance where a crime is alleged or there exists evidence that a crime occurred. Make an arrest in every legally mandated instance.
   - Refer every domestic violence investigation with prima facie evidence of criminal misconduct to the appropriate prosecuting agency in a timely manner.
   - Do not discontinue domestic violence investigations merely because the victim recants or indicates unwillingness to testify in disciplinary hearings.
   - Mandate termination of employees in serious cases of domestic violence where officers demonstrate by a convincing pattern that they cannot control their abusive conduct.
   - Increase suspensions for sustained acts of domestic violence in length and severity. Mete out long-term suspensions or terminations to those who have repeated instances of sustained allegations.
   - Document sustained allegations of misconduct and consider them in performance reviews and promotions.
   - Develop an Anti–Domestic Violence Program under the direction of the Psychologist. Require contracts to include mandatory counselling in all sustained complaints involving domestic violence.

Alcohol/Drug Abuse

8. Although most police services have addressed unsatisfactory work performance that includes, but is not limited to, alcohol/drug abuse, we recommend that the Psychological Services Section in an ongoing manner review this policy and procedure. (Alcoholism is a major risk factor.)

Professional and Ethical Challenges

9. Police services must be sensitive to professional and ethical dilemmas that suicide and homicide-suicide present if we are going to prevent a future one. This will require a balance between privacy and prevention, without enabling blue walls. Understandably, police officers should not

avoid or keep secrets from others about fellow officers' risks for suicide or homicide. There should be a clear mandate to not buy into a suicidogenic barrier such as dissembling. It will require cooperation of police services staff, not only the officers, but all of us.

INTERVENTION

II This is primary and here we follow the ecological model, understanding and thus preventing and controlling suicide and homicide-suicide at the individual, relationship, community, and societal levels (Dahlberg & Krug, 2002). Intervention relates to the treatment and care of a suicidal and suicidal-homicidal crisis or suicidal (homicidal-suicidal) problems at all levels (Leenaars, 2004). We first present a few general and then specific recommendations. We subdivided the recommendations into the following: Intervention: General; Mental Health Services (especially high risk officers); Assessment (of recruits and ongoing); Specialized Programs (such as women issues in policing); and finally, the controversial, Gun Control.

Intervention: General

10. First and foremost, we recommend that the Psychologist along with peer support staff be assigned responsibilities in intervention.
11. Many officers can serve as life-saving agents; nonetheless, professionally trained people, psychiatrists, psychologists, social workers, psychiatric nurses, crisis workers, and so on, continue to play the primary roles in intervention. Thus, although equally true for prevention and postvention, intervention will call for the ongoing development of community and social linkages.

Mental Health Services for Staff. High Risk Officers

12. Healthy police services contribute to the overall wellness of individuals' psychological health and resilience by reinforcing fair practices and open communication among all levels of the service.
13. To help officers (and we imply all staff) take the first difficult step to intervention, the police service should develop and increase accessibility to confidential health and mental health services; this is paramount. Essentially, officers need a safe place out of administrative view to go for help. The Psychologist will be essential; however, it is necessary to establish a network of psychiatrists, psychologists, and other mental health workers in the community who are familiar with police problems. Therefore, when troubled members are in need of such service, they can be referred easily.

14. We recommend that, with police associations, a list of clinicians in the community with experience with police be developed based on the input of the officers. This list should be recompiled on an ongoing basis and be readily available to officers. (We have learned of suicidogenic errors, when lists are only updated every 6 months; it must be ongoing, based on all officers' feedback.)
15. Police services should support easy access to psychological, medical, and other empirically based interventions. This again should address blue walls, stigma, and other barriers to help-seeking, a major deterrent worldwide in officers getting help; but not only officers. It is a common problem, not unique to police.
16. Police services should develop criteria to identify and track high risk officers (such as officers with marital/intimate partner difficulties, alcohol/substance abuse, work problems, traumatization and other life problems) so that timely support can be provided. The Psychologist should work with supervisory personnel to identify and review when officers are possibly at risk for emotional disturbance, suicide, and homicide-suicide.

Assessment

17. Police services need to develop and implement a comprehensive psychological assessment in recruiting. This screen is already a major aspect of most police departments. We highly encourage a review, however (for example, periodic reassessment as part of the prescribed standard operating procedure (SOP) to assure that wellness prevails). We recognize the limits of psychological testing, due to the low base rate and complexity of events like suicide and homicide-suicide in officers; yet predisposing personality factors (depression) and precipitating family history (family violence, substance abuse) can be evaluated. We highly endorse a comprehensive assessment, which includes but is not limited to the Minnesota Multiphasic Personality Inventory-2 (MMPI-2), with inclusion of the revised clinical scales (Selbom, Fischler, & Ben-Porth, 2007). The latter scales are most effective in screening a wide array of risks.
18. Police services should undertake periodic reassessment as part of the prescribed SOP to assure that wellness prevails. We recommend that police services establish a clear process of reassessment. Within a more comprehensive approach to evaluation, this must include psychological reassessment; reassessment of officers assigned to at-risk for traumatization, such as Administration, Major Crime Division, Child Pornography, Gang Unit, Emergency Response Unit, to provide a few examples, not a complete list.

19. Psychological assessment presupposes an effective, nonstigmatized referral system for dealing with affairs in psychological disturbance, often ones that are normal, not "crazy," given the very nature of the job. PTSD is very common, in fact. This is necessary so that any problems observed can receive appropriate treatment in a supportive atmosphere.

Specialized Programs

20. Police services can do much, not only in intervention, but also in educating their officers to understand and to promote help-seeking for police stress, despair, and suicide. We recommend that the Psychologist, with the peer support officers, develop such programs with other community individuals/agencies.
21. In addition to the above services, police services within the larger community should develop programs in the following areas:
    - Family/intimate partner involvement: Seminars should be given to police recruits and their families/partners so they understand the effects of police work. Counselling services must be made available, with community liaison to families/partners and officers.
    - Stress awareness: Stress awareness is a sound method to help individuals. By the very nature of their job, police are placed at risk for stress, but also to avoidance and dissembling. Thus, a well-rounded stress-education program should include identification of stress, the value and techniques of physical exercise, benefits of proper nutrition, interpersonal communication and coping style.
    - Retirement counselling: Retirement can be a difficult phase for most officers. Retirement counselling should be enhanced, if requested.
    - Women in policing: Seminars should be provided and enhanced in awareness, training, and policies to the unique demands facing female police officers in a male-dominated police profession.

    We do not see this list as exhaustive, but a beginning to develop wellness programs beyond the individual level.

Gun Control

22. Beyond the individual and relationship level, we would recommend the following, specifically on gun control:

    We recognize that police services across the United States and Canada clearly spell out in their policies and procedures for the safe storage, discharge, handling, and transportation of firearms. We do not advocate further gun control, such as disarming officers, except for the enforcement of those in law already. These laws, together with most effective policies and procedures in police services, given our own expertise on the topic (Leenaars, 2007), are sufficient, if followed. Yet, we would like to note a few recommendations.

- Like all citizens, police officers are subject to laws; this includes restriction of firearms due to mental health condition. Officers with specified severe emotional disturbance are prohibited from gun access. Psychopathology is, based on research, a primary factor in risk. Officers with alcohol/substance abuse are prohibited from gun access. Officers at risk for suicide or homicide are by law forbidden to have gun access. This is not simply our recommendation but it is also the law in the United States and Canada. The Psychologist will be essential in evaluation of such disturbances and risks, but it also requires the support of the entire community.
- Gun laws require review and evaluation of disclosure of risk by family or intimate partners; thus, all complaints must be assessed/reviewed and proper actions taken if warranted.
- As already noted, officers charged with domestic violence may not have access to guns; again, this is the law.
- Waiting periods are shown to be effective; we recommend that appropriate waiting periods are undertaken before access to guns is again provided to officers previously identified as at-risk. This is in keeping with the evidence-based fact that psychotherapy, medication, and so on can be effective. The Psychologist, with community liaison, must determine each individual's ability to have access, not by a general policy alone.
- Despite the efforts of the Psychologist and administration of police services, there has been, and will be problems due to the availability of guns. (How did Lt. Michael Pigott get the gun from his partner's locker?) We recommend ongoing review of availability/access, and ongoing training, but also communication about dissembling/masking in officers. Risks must be addressed immediately; yet as the literature on gun control shows, environmental control works better than people control. Thus, environmental methods must be undertaken if and when necessary.

POSTVENTION

III Postvention refers to those things done after the event has occurred, the traumatic after-effects. In the case of police suicide, these refer not only to family, friends, and fellow officers, but probably the entire community. (How did the community react to Chief Thomas Moffatt's suicide?) Here we offer some general policies and strategies; we recommend that the

Psychological Services Section, with the peer support officers, together with community experts, develop comprehensive efforts.

Postvention: General

23. It is recommended that in collaboration and cooperation with local Survivor and Bereavement services, that police services strongly support community programs for survivors. Yet police services, with the same groups, also need to develop their own postvention program, not only for suicides, but also for other trauma in police services (such as murder of an officer or suicide by cop). At the very least, the strategies should include consultation, crisis intervention, community linkage, assessment and psychotherapy, education, liaison with the media, and follow-up.
24. Although we wish to stress that postventions are not solely the responsibility of the police services, police services can at least develop some major steps toward postvention. Following Loo (2001), these include the following:
    - Establish and execute your standing operating procedure for postvention policies and procedures. The procedures should specify the key positions/persons responsible for initiating the procedures. For example, the immediate supervisor, the officer who first hears about the suicide (e.g., the duty officer), the services' Psychologist, and Internal Affairs.
    - Have a crisis team trained and ready to have a planning meeting to initiate the plan. The team could be a mix of health professionals and trained peer counselors, both police services and community based.
    - Notify the departmental administration; next-of-kin; family physician; clergy, if known; and other key persons.
    - A departmental communication release should be made as soon as practical to let fellow officers and staffs know the facts rather than have the grapevine circulate rumors. Manage the external media by having a timely press release so that facts rather than myths reach the media.
    - Have a carefully picked debriefing facility readily available. While it may be practical to use a room in a police facility, an off-site facility such as a meeting or conference room in a community center might be better for the survivors.
    - Do at least one follow-up session to address unresolved concerns and any new issues that arose since the debriefing. Debriefing, of course, is not sufficient for at-risk officers; they need longer-term intervention.
    - Conduct a confidential evaluation of the postvention by having participants complete, for example, a confidential and anonymous evaluation questionnaire a week or two after the debriefing to identify particularly

what worked well and what needs to be improved for future postvention. Alternatively, the evaluation might be conducted as a group session thus allowing for interactions among survivors but precluding anonymity.

CONCLUDING REMARKS

We need to continue to develop a multidimensional or ecological approach to understanding suicide—and the suicide of that individual, such as of the 93 officers in the 1930s great suicide epidemic in New York, Lt. Michael Pigott, Chief Thomas Moffatt, and Inspector Kelly Johnson—that can be made useful and life saving. The same is true for homicide-suicide. No one likely predicted those officers' suicide or homicide-suicide, maybe some of the NY officers. Some left clues, whereas most dissembled. There were and are *blue walls*. How could we reach through the *Othello* mask? What would have helped? What prevention efforts could be in place to reduce the risks of future incidents? The deaths could have probably been prevented, although despite even the best efforts, there will be casualties. There is no perfection in *prevention*, only life-saving efforts. What intervention (psychotherapy, peer support program, healing circle, medication, gun control, and so on) will effectively work with that officer? What postvention efforts need to be in place? We need to not only be evidenced-based, but also officer-centered. We need to know what we are talking about, investigating, and treating. Thus it follows: What do police officers know? What would they recommend? What would the peer-support officers recommend? They are the experts on police, not us. Yet we believe that the general recommendations herein should be reviewed and can be easily followed, maybe with this or that specific modification under the model a police service chooses to establish. There is no cookbook here either, only our good will, something Gregory Zilboorg called for in 1940 (actually in the beginning in July 1938) in New York. Zilboorg had, in fact, a therapeutic relationship with many officers, the New York police service, and the community. The epidemic in the 1930s in New York was stopped. Can we do the same? Indeed, this is our aim. We hope that this book will be effective in preventing suicide among suicidal police officers and homicidal-suicidal police officers, the very request of the great American political hero, the would-be United States senator, Mayor Fiorello La Guardia. In 1938, La Guardia recommended the most famous New York investigations in police suicide, *a psychological autopsy*. He afforded "every cooperation" to the understanding of the suicides and made sure that "a very useful purpose" was made of every one of Zilboorg's and his team's recommendations. There was not only understanding (some 4,000 triple-spaced typewritten pages) but also policies and procedures implemented at prediction and control. In 1940 in New York, La Guardia, Zilboorg, officers, and many more people worked together. There was *perseverance*. There were implemented recommendations, much the same as ours (J. S. Mill's method of agreement.) There was much that was done in New York, but more could have been done, especially for survivors. That is often true; the main point was that mental health, and specifically suicide *prevention* policy and procedure were developed and implemented. Suicides were prevented. Police services can do so today. We need a La Guardia. We need a Zilboorg. We need all of us. We can save officers lives. We need an *ecological* approach. Or will we continue to allow our officers to die by suicide?

References

Aamoldt, M., & Stalnakar, N. (2001). Police officer suicide: Frequency and officer profiles. In D. Sheehan & J. Warren (Eds.), *Suicide & law enforcement* (pp. 383–398). Washington, DC: FBI.

Adjacic-Gross, V., Killias, M., Hepp, U., Gadola, E., Bapp, M., Lauber, C. et al. (2006). Changing times: A longitudinal analysis of international firearm suicide data. *American Journal of Public Health, 96,* 1752–1755.

Allen, N. (1980). *Homicide*. New York: Human Sciences Press.

Allen, N. (1983). Homicide followed by suicide: Los Angeles, 1970–1979. *Suicide & Life-Threatening Behavior, 13,* 155–165.

Allen, N. (1993). Murder among elderly Anglo females. In. A. Leenaars (Ed.), *Suicidology: Essays in honor of Edwin S. Shneidman* (pp. 93–104). Northvale, NJ: Jason Aronson, Inc.

Allport, G. (1942). *The use of personal documents in psychological science*. New York: Social Science Research Council.

Allport, G. (1962). The general and the unique in psychological science. *Journal of Personality, 30,* 405–422.

American Psychiatric Association. (1994). *Diagnostic and statistical manual of mental disorders* (4th ed.). Washington, DC: Author.

American Psychiatric Association. (2003). Practice guidelines for the assessment and treatment of patients with suicidal behavior. *Supplement to the American Journal of Psychiatry, 160*(11), 1–183.

Andrews, L. (1996a). *Suicide in the RCMP: 1984 to 1995*. Ottawa: Royal Canadian Mounted Police.

Andrews, L. (1996b). *A cross national comparison of police suicide rates*. Ottawa: Royal Canadian Mounted Police.

Asberg, M., Traskman, L., & Thorien, P. (1976). 5-H1AA in cerebrospinal fluid: A biochemical suicide prediction? *Archives of General Psychiatry, 33,* 1193–1197.

Ayer, A. (Ed.). (1959). *Logical positivism*. New York: Free Press.

Baker, T., & Baker, J. (1996). Preventing police suicide. *FBI Law Enforcement Bulletin, October,* 24–27.

Barak, A., & Miran, O. (2005). Writing characteristics of suicidal people on the Internet: A psychological investigation of emerging social environments. *Suicide & Life-Threatening Behavior, 35,* 507–524.

Barnes, J. (2007). Murder followed by suicide in Australia, 1973–1992: A research note. *Journal of Sociology, 36,* 1–14.

Barraclough, B. (1986). Illness and suicide. In J. Morgan (Ed.), *Suicide: Helping those at risk* (pp. 61–69). London: King's College.

Barraclough, B., & Harris, E. (2002). Suicide preceded by murder: The epidemiology of homicide-suicide in England and Wales 1988–92. *Psychological Medicine, 32,* 577–584.

Barrett, K. (1997). Police suicide: Is anyone listening? *Journal of Safe Management of Disruptive and Assaultive Behaviour, 5,* 6–9.

Beautrais, A., Fergusson, D., & Horwood, L. (2006). Firearms legislation and reduction in firearms-related suicide deaths in New Zealand. *Australian and New Zealand Journal of Psychiatry, 40,* 253–259.

Beck, A. (1976). *Cognitive therapy and emotional disorders.* New York: International University Press.

Beck, A., & Freeman, A. (Eds.). (1990). *Cognitive therapy of personality disorders.* New York: Guilford Press.

Beck, A., Kovacs, M., & Weissman, A. (1975). Hopelessness and suicidal behavior: An overview. *Journal of the American Medical Association, 234*, 1146–1149.

Beck, A., Resnick, H., & Lettieri, D. (Eds.). (1974). *The prediction of suicide.* Bowie, MD: Charles Press.

Berg, A., Hem, E., Lau, B., & Ekeberg, Ø. (2006). Help-seeking in the Norwegian police service. *Journal of Occupational Health, 48,* 145–153.

Berg, A., Hem, E., Lau, B., Loeb, M., & Ekeberg, Ø. (2003). Suicidal ideation and attempts in Norwegian police. *Suicide & Life-Threatening Behavior, 33,* 302–312.

Bergin, A., & Lambert, M. (1978). The evaluation of therapeutic outcome. In S. Garfield & A. Bergin (Eds.), *Handbook of psychotherapy and behavior change: An empirical analysis* (2nd ed., pp. 139–189). Chichester, UK: John Wiley & Sons.

Berman, A. (1979). Dyadic death: Murder-suicide. *Suicide & Life-Threatening Behavior, 9,* 15–23.

Berman, A., & Jobes, D. (1991). *Adolescent suicide: Assessment and intervention.* Washington, DC: American Psychological Association Press.

Bertolote, J. (Ed.). (1993). *Guidelines for the primary prevention of mental, neurological and psychosocial disorders: Suicide.* Geneva: World Health Organization.

Beutler, L., Malik, M., Alimohamed, S., Harwood, T., Talebi, H., Noble, S., et al. (2004). Therapist variables. In M. Lambert (Ed.), *Bergin and Garfield's handbook of psychotherapy and behavior change* (5th ed., pp. 227–306). New York: John Wiley & Sons.

Bongar, B. (1991). *The suicidal patient: Clinical and legal standards of care.* Washington, DC: American Psychological Association.

Bongar, B., & Greaney, S. (1994). Essential clinical and legal issues when working with the suicidal patient. In A. Leenaars, J. Maltsberger, & R. Neimeyer (Eds.), *Treatment of suicidal people* (pp. 179–194). Washington, DC: Taylor & Francis.

Bossarte, R., Sion, T., & Barker, L. (2007, September). Characteristics of homicide followed by suicide incidents in multiple states, 2003–04. *Injury Prevention, 12,* ii33–ii36.

Bostwick, J. (2000). Affective disorders and suicide risk: A re-examination. *American Journal of Psychiatry, 157*, 1925–1932.

Bourdouris, J. (1974). A classification of homicides. *Criminology, 11,* 525–556.

Brent, D. (1989). The psychological autopsy: Methodological considerations for the study of adolescent suicide. *Suicide & Life-Threatening Behavior, 19*, 43–57.

Brent, D. (1992, April). *Psychiatric effects of exposure to suicide among friends and acquaintances*. Paper presented at the conference of the American Association of Suicidology, Chicago.

Brent, D., Perper, J., Moritz, G., Baugher, M., Schweers, J., & Roth, C. (1993). Firearms and adolescent suicide. *American Journal of Diseases of Children, 147,* 1066–1071.

Bronfenbrenner, U. (1979). *The ecology of human development: Experts by nature and design*. Cambridge, MA: Harvard University Press.

Bronisch, T., Wolfersdorf, M., & Leenaars, A. (Eds.). (2005). Suicidality, bipolar disorders & psychopharmacology. *Archives of Suicide Research, 9,* 231–319.

Buteau, J., Lesage, A., & Kiely, M. (1993). Homicide followed by suicide: A Quebec case series, 1988–1990. *Canadian Journal of Psychiatry, 38,* 552–556.

Canada's Standing Committee on Social Affairs, Science & Terminology. (2006). *Out of the shadow at last*. Ottawa: Government of Canada.

Canetto, S. (1994). Gender issues in the treatment of suicidal individuals. In A. Leenaars, J. Maltsberger, & R. Neimeyer (Eds.), *Treatment of suicidal people* (pp. 115–126). Washington, DC: Taylor and Francis.

Canetto, S., & Lester, D. (Eds.). (1995). *Women and suicidal behavior*. New York: Springer.

Caplan, G. (1964). *Principles of preventive psychiatry*. New York: Basic Books.

Carnap, R. (1959). Psychology in physical language. In A. Ayer (Ed.), *Logical positivism* (pp. 165–197). New York: Free Press (Original work published 1931.)

Carr, J. (2001). Suicide of a chief executive officer: Implications for intervention. In D. Sheehan & J. Warren (Eds.), *Suicide and law enforcement* (pp. 67–70). Washington, DC: FBI.

Carrington, P., & Moyer, S. (1994a). Gun control and suicide in Ontario. *American Journal of Psychiatry, 151,* 606–608.

Carrington, P., & Moyer, S. (1994b). Gun availability and suicide in Canada. *Studies on Crime and Crime Prevention, 3,* 168–178.

Chavez, A., Paramo-Castillo, D., Leenaars, A., & Leenaars, L. (2006). Suicide notes in Mexico: What do they tell us? *Suicide and Life-Threatening Behavior, 36,* 709–715.

Chavez-Hernandez, A., Leenaars, A., Chavez-de Sanchez, M., & Leenaars, L. (2009). Suicide notes from Mexico and the United States: A thematic analysis. *Salud Publico de Mexico, 51,* 314–320. [In Spanish]

Clark, J. (1977). Police careers may take a beating from fed domestic violence. *Law Enforcement News, xxiii,* 1–3.

Clark, S., & Goldney, R. (1995). Grief reactions and recovery in a support group for people bereaved by suicide. *Crisis, 16,* 27–33.

Conroy, D. (2001). Developing a plan: Helping a department heal after a police suicide. In D. Sheehan & J. Warren (Eds.), *Suicide and law enforcement* (pp. 71–81). Washington, DC: FBI.

Cormier, B., Augliker, C., Boyer, R., Kennedy, M., & Mersereau, G. (1971). The psychodynamics of homicide committed in a specific relationship. *Canadian Journal of Criminology and Corrections, 13,* 1–8.

Cummings, P., Koepsell, T., Grossman, D., Savarino, J., & Thompson, R. (1997). The association between the purchase of a handgun and homicide and suicide. *American Journal of Public Health, 87,* 974–978.

Curphey, T. (1967). The forensic pathologist and the multidisciplinary approach to death. In E. Shneidman (Ed.), *Essays in self-destruction* (pp. 463–474). New York: Science House.

Dahlberg, L., & Krug, E. (2002). Violence—A global public health problem. In WHO (Ed.), *World report on violence and health* (pp. 3–21). Geneva: World Health Organization.

Danto, B. (1978). Police suicide. *Police stress, 1,* 32–40.

Danto, B. (1979). New frontiers in the relationship between suicidology and law enforcement. *Suicide & Life-Threatening Behavior, 9,* 195–205.

de Boismont, B. (1856). *Du suicide et la folie suicide.* Paris: Germer Bailliere.

Demirel, B., Akar, T., Sayin, A., Candansayar, S., & Leenaars, A. (2008). Farewell to the world: Suicide notes from Turkey. *Suicide and Life-Threatening Behavior, 38,* 122–127.

Department of Health, UK. (2002). *National suicide prevention strategy for England.* London: Author.

Department of Justice, Canada (1996). *A statistical analysis of the impacts of the 1977 firearms control legislation.* Ottawa: Department of Justice.

Diamond, G., More, D., Hawkins, A., & Soucar, E. (1995). Comment on Black's (1993) article "Comparing genuine and simulated suicide notes: A new perspective." *Journal of Consulting and Clinical Psychology, 63*, 46–48.

Dogra, T., Leenaars, A., Raintji, R., Lalwani, S., Girdhar, S., Wenckstern, S., et al. (2007). Menstruation and suicide: An exploratory study. *Psychological Reports, 101,* 430–434.

Donaldson, D., Spirito, A., & Overholser, J. (2003). Treatment of adolescent suicide attempters. In A. Spirito & J. Overholser (Eds.), *Evaluating and treating adolescent suicide attempters: From research to practice* (pp. 295–321). New York: Academic Press.

Douglas, J. (1967). *The social meaning of suicide.* New Jersey: Princeton University Press.

Dowling, F., & Monynihan, G. (2004). Suicide among police. Letter to the editor. *American Journal of Psychiatry, 161,* 767.

Durkheim, E. (1951). *Suicide* (J. Spaulding & G. Simpson, Trans.). Glencoe, IL: The Free Press. (Original work published 1897.)

Easteal, P. (1994). Homicides-suicides between adult sexual intimates: An Australian study. *Suicide & Life-Threatening Behavior, 24,* 140–151.

Etzersdorfer, E., Kapusta, N., & Sonneck, G. (2006). Suicide by shooting is correlated to rate of gun licenses in Austrian counties. *Wiener Klinische Wochenschrift, 118,* 464–468.

Exner, J. (1986). *The Rorschach: A comprehensive system* (2nd ed., Vol. 1). New York: Wiley.

Ex-officer sues over Mayerthorpe. (2009, March 13). *The Windsor Star,* p. A11.

Farberow, N. (Ed.). (1980). *The many faces of suicide*. New York: McGraw-Hill.

Fawcett, J. (1997). The detection and consequences of anxiety in clinical depression. *Journal of Clinical Psychiatry, 58*(Suppl. 8), 35–40.

Felthouse, A., Hempel, A., Heredia, A., Freeman, E., Goodness, K., Holzer, C., et al. (2001). Combined homicide-suicide in Galveston County. *Journal of Forensic Sciences, 46,* 586–592.

Ferri, E. (1917). *Criminal sociology*. Boston: Little, Brown.

Fishbain, D. (1994). Homicide followed by suicide [Letter to the editor]. *Canadian Journal of Psychiatry, 39,* 385–386.

Fishbain, D. (2003). Letter to the editor. *Psychological Medicine, 33,* 375.

Fishbain, D., Rao, V., & Aldrich, T. (1985). Female homicide-suicide perpetrators: A controlled study. *Journal of Forensic Sciences, 30,* 1148–1156.

Foster, T. (2003). Suicide note themes and suicide prevention. *International Journal of Psychiatry in Medicine, 33*, 323–331.

Frank, J., Gliedman, L., Imber, S., Nash, E., & Stone, A. (1957). Why patients leave psychotherapy. *American Medical Association, 77,* 283–299.

Frederick, C. (1969, March). Suicide notes: A survey and evaluation. *Bulletin of Suicidology,* 27–32.

Freedheim, D. (Ed.). (1992). *History of psychotherapy*. Washington, DC: American Psychological Association.

Freud, S. (1974). Psychopathology of everyday life. In J. Strachey (Ed. & Trans.), *The standard edition of the complete psychological works of Sigmund Freud* (Vol. VI, pp. 1–310). London: Hogarth Press (Original work published 1901.)

Freud, S. (1974). Analytic therapy. In J. Strachey (Ed. & Trans.), *The standard edition of the complete psychological works of Sigmund Freud* (Vol. XVI, pp. 448–463). London: Hogarth Press. (Original work published 1916.)

Freud, S. (1974). Mourning and melancholia. In J. Strachey (Ed.), *The standard edition of the complete psychological works of Sigmund Freud* (Vol. XIV, pp. 239–260). London: Hogarth. (Original work published 1917a.)

Freud, S. (1974). General theory of neurosis. In J. Strachey (Ed. & Trans.), *The standard edition of the complete psychological works of Sigmund Freud* (Vol. XVI, pp. 243–483). London: Hogarth Press. (Original work published 1917b.)

Freud, S. (1974). A case of homosexuality in a woman. In J. Strachey (Ed. & Trans.), *The standard edition of the complete psychological works of Sigmund Freud* (Vol. XVII, pp. 147–172). London: Hogarth Press. (Original work published 1920.)

Freud, S. (1974). Group psychology and the analysis of the ego. In J. Strachey (Ed. & Trans.), *The standard edition of the complete psychological works of Sigmund Freud* (Vol. XVIII, pp. 67–147). London: Hogarth Press. (Original work published 1921.)

Freud, S. (1974). The economic problem of masochism. In J. Strachey (Ed. & Trans.), *The standard edition of the complete psychological works of Sigmund Freud* (Vol. XIX or 19I, pp. 157–170). London: Hogarth Press. (Original work published 1924.)

Friedman, P. (1967a). Suicide among police: A study of ninety-three suicides among New York policemen, 1934–1940. In E. Shneidman (Ed.), *Essays in self-destruction* (pp. 415–449). New York: Jason Aronson, Inc.

Friedman, P. (Ed.). (1967b). *On suicide*. New York: International Universities Press. (Original work published 1910.)

Garbarino, J., & Crouter, A. (1978). Defining the community context for child-parent relations: The correlations of child maltreatment. *Child Development, 49*, 604–616.

Garfield, S., & Bergin, A. (Eds.). (1978). *Handbook of psychotherapy and behavior change: An empirical analysis* (2nd ed.). Chichester, UK: John Wiley & Sons.

Garrison, C., Lewinsohn, P., Marsteller, F., Langhinrichsen, J., & Lann, I. (1991). The assessment of suicidal behavior in adolescents. *Suicide & Life-Threatening Behavior, 21*, 217–230.

Gaska, C. (1980). *The rate of suicide, potential for suicide, and recommendations for prevention among retired police officers.* Doctoral dissertation. Detroit, MI: Wayne State University.

Geberth, V. (1993, July). Suicide by cop. *Law and Order,* pp. 105–107.

Girdhar, S., Leenaars, A., Dogra, T. D., Leenaars, L., & Kumar, G. (2004). Suicide notes in India: What do they tell us? *Archives of Suicide Research, 8*, 179–185.

Goffman, E. (1974). *Frame analysis*. New York: Harper Colophon.

Goldblatt, M. (1992). *Richard Cory suicides: Diagnostic questions.* Paper presented at the annual conference of the American Association of Suicidology, Chicago.

Goldney, R. (1979). Medical responsibility in murder and suicide. *Medical Journal of Australia, 1,* 50–59.

Hadley, S., & Strupp, H. (1976). Contemporary views of negative effects in psychotherapy: An integrated account. *Archives of General Psychiatry, 33,* 1291–1302.

Hahn, R., Bilukha, O., Crosby, A., Fullilove, M., Liberman, A., Moscicki, E., et al. (2003, October 3). First reports evaluating the effectiveness of strategies for preventing violence: Firearms laws. *MMWR. Morbidity and Mortality Weekly Report, 52,* 11–20.

Harper, D., & Voigt, L. (2007). Homicide followed by suicide: An integrated theoretical perspective. *Homicide Studies, 11,* 293–318.

Hawton, K., & van Heeringen, C. (Eds.). (2000). *Suicide and attempted suicide*. Chichester, UK: John Wiley & Sons.

Hem, E., Berg, A., & Ekeberg, Ø. (2004). Suicide among police [Letter to the editor]. *American Journal of Psychiatry, 161,* 767–76.

Hempel, C. (1966). *Philosophy of natural sciences*. Englewood Cliffs, NJ: Prentice-Hall, Inc.

Hendin, H., Haas, A., Maltsberger, J., Koestner, B., & Szanto, K. (2006). Problems in psychotherapy with suicidal patients. *American Journal of Psychiatry, 163,* 67–72.

Hendin, H., Haas, A., Maltsberger, J., Szanto, K., & Rabinowicz, H. (2004). Factors contributing to therapists' distress after a suicide of a patient. *American Journal of Psychiatry, 161,* 1442–1446.

Henry, A., & Short, J. (1954). *Suicide and homicide*. New York: Free Press.

Ho, T., Yip, P., Chiu, C., & Halliday, P. (1998). Suicide notes: What do they tell us? *Acta Psychiatrica Scandinavica, 98*, 467–473.

Hoch, P. (1972). *Differential diagnosis in clinical psychiatry: The lectures of Paul H. Hoch, M.D.* M. Strahl & N. Lewis (Eds.). New York: Science House.

Hollon, S., & Fawcett, J. (2001). Combined medication and psychotherapy. In G. Gabbard (Ed.), *Treatments of psychiatric disorders* (Vol. 2, pp. 1247–1266). Washington, DC: American Psychiatric Publication, Inc.

Horvitz, L. (1994, November 7). Can police solve their epidemic of suicide? *Insight,* 9–12. http://www.massey.ac.nz/~trauma1

Hughes, S., & Neimeyer, R. (1990). A cognitive model of suicidal behavior. In D. Lester (Ed.), *Current concepts of suicide* (pp. 1–28). Philadelphia: The Charles Press.

Husserl, E. (1973). *The idea of phenomenology* (W. Alston & G. Nokhnikian, Trans.). The Hague: Martinus Nijhoff. (Original work published 1907.)

Hutson, H., Anglin, D., Yarbrough, J., Hardaway, J., Russell, M., Strote, J., et al. (1998). Suicide by cop. *Annals of Emergency Medicine, 32,* 665–669.

International Association of Chiefs of Police. (2003). *A policy of the IACP police response to violence against women project*. Washington, DC: Author.

Ivanoff, A. (1994). *The New York City police suicide training project* (pp. 5–15). New York: Police Foundation.

James, W. (1890). *The principles of psychology*. New York: Henry Holt & Co.

Jenkins, R., McCulloch, A., Friedli, C., & Parker, C. (2002). *Developing a national mental health policy*. East Sussex, UK: Psychological Press Ltd.

Jenkins, R., & Singh, B. (2000). General population strategies of suicide prevention. In K. Hawton & K. van Heeringen (Eds.), *The international handbook of suicide and attempted suicide* (pp. 597–615). Chichester, UK: John Wiley & Sons.

Johnson, H., & Hotton, T. (2003). Losing control. *Homicide Studies, 7,* 58–84.

Kahane, H. (1973). *Logic and philosophy* (2nd ed.). Belmont, CA: Wadsworth Publishing House Co. Inc.

Kamerman, J. (1993). The illegacy of suicide. In A. Leenaars (Ed.), *Suicidology: Essays in honor of Edwin S. Shneidman* (pp. 346–355). Northvale, NJ: Jason Aronson, Inc.

Kamerman, J. (2001). The social construction of police and correctional officer suicide. In D. Sheehan & J. Warren (Eds.), *Suicide and law enforcement* (pp. 529–538). Washington, DC: FBI.

Kellerman, A., Rivara, F., Somes, G., Reay, D., Francisco, J., Banton, J., et al. (1992). Suicide in the home in relation to gun ownership. *New England Journal of Medicine, 327,* 467–472.

Kennedy, D., Homant, R., & Hupp, R. (1998, August). Suicide by cop. *FBI Law Enforcement Bulletin,* 7.

Kerlinger, F. (1964). *Foundations of behavioral research*. New York: Holt, Rinehart & Winston, Inc.

Kernberg, O. (1973). Summary and conclusion of "Psychotherapy and psychoanalysis: Final report of the Menninger Foundation's Psychotherapy Research Project." *International Journal of Psychiatry, 11,* 62–77.

Knizek, B., & Hjelmeland, H. (2007). A theoretical model for interpreting suicidal behavior as communication. *Theory & Psychology, 17*, 697–720.

Kuhn, T. (1962). *The structure of scientific revolutions*. Chicago: University of Chicago Press.

Lambert, M. (Ed.). (2004). *Bergin and Garfield's handbook of psychotherapy and behavior change* (5th ed.). New York: John Wiley & Sons.

Lambert, M., & Bergin, A. (1992). Achievements and limitations of psychotherapy research. In D. Freedheim (Ed.), *History of psychotherapy* (pp. 360–390). Washington, DC: American Psychological Association.

Lambert, M., Bergin, A., & Garfield, S. (2004). Introduction and historical overview. In M. Lambert (Ed.), *Bergin and Garfield's handbook of psychotherapy and behavior change* (5th ed., pp. 3–15). New York: John Wiley & Sons.

Lambert, M., & Ogles, B. (2004). The efficacy and effectiveness of psychotherapy. In M. Lambert (Ed.), *Bergin and Garfield's handbook of psychotherapy and behavior change* (5th ed., pp. 139–193). New York: John Wiley & Sons.

Lazarus, A. (1971). *Behavior therapy & beyond.* New York: McGraw-Hill.

Leenaars, A. (1988). *Suicide Notes*. New York: Human Sciences Press.

Leenaars, A. (1989). Suicide across the adult life-span: An archival study. *Crisis, 10,* 132–151.

Leenaars, A. (1992). Suicide notes from Canada and United States. *Perceptual and Motor Skills, 74*, 278.

Leenaars, A. (Ed.). (1993a). *Suicidology: Essays in honor of Edwin S. Shneidman*. Northvale, NJ: Jason Aronson, Inc.

Leenaars, A. (1993b). Unconscious processes. In A. Leenaars (Ed.), *Suicidology: Essays in honor of Edwin S. Shneidman* (pp. 127–147). Northvale, NJ: Aronson.

Leenaars, A. (1995). Clinical evaluation of suicide risk. *Psychiatry and Clinical Neurosciences, 49*(Suppl. 1), 561–568.

Leenaars, A. (1996). Suicide: A multidimensional malaise. *Suicide & Life-Threatening Behavior, 26*, 221–236.

Leenaars, A. (1997). Rick: A suicide of a young adult. *Suicide & Life-Threatening Behavior, 27*, 15–27.

Leenaars, A. (Ed.). (1999a). *Lives and deaths: Selections from the works of Edwin S. Shneidman*. Philadelphia: Brunner/Mazel.

Leenaars, A. (1999b). Suicide notes in the courtroom. *Journal of Clinical Forensic Medicine, 6,* 39–48.

Leenaars, A. (2002, May 30). The people vs Guy Leslie Barker. Certified for publication in the court of appeal of the state of California, Fourth Appellate District, Division Three. G028224 (Superior Ct. No. 00NF0451) Opinion.

Leenaars, A. (2004). *Psychotherapy with suicidal people*. Chichester, UK: John Wiley & Sons.

Leenaars, A. (2006). Psychotherapy with suicidal people: The commonalities. *Archives of Suicide Research, 10,* 305–322.

Leenaars, A. (2007). Gun-control legislation and the impact on suicide. *Crisis, 28,* 50–57.

Leenaars, A. (2008). Suicide: A cross-cultural theory. In F. Leong & M. Leach (Eds.), *Suicide among racial and ethnic minority groups* (pp. 13–37). New York: Routledge.

Leenaars, A. (2009a). Death systems and suicide around the world. In J. Morgan, P. Laungani, & S. Palmer (Eds.), *Death and bereavement around the world* (Vol. 5, pp. 103–138). Amityville, NY: Baywood.

Leenaars, A. (2009b). Controlling the availability of means of suicide—Gun availability and control. In D. Wasserman & C. Wasserman (Eds.), *The Oxford textbook of suicidology and suicide prevention: A global perspective* (pp. 577–581). Oxford, UK: Oxford University Press.

Leenaars, A. (in press). Evidence-based psychotherapy with suicidal people: A systematic review. In M. Pompili & R. Tatarelli (Eds.), *Evidence-based practice in suicide prevention: A source book.* Gottingen, Germany: Horafe & Huber.

Leenaars, A., & Balance, W. (1984). A logical empirical approach to the study of suicide notes. *Canadian Journal of Behavioural Science, 16*, 248–256.

Leenaars, A., Balance, W., Pellarin, S., Aversano, G., Magli, A., & Wenckstern, S. (1988). Facts and myths of suicide in Canada. *Death Studies, 12*, 191–210.

Leenaars, A., Cantor, C., Connolly, J., EchoHawk, M., Gailiene, D., He, Z., et al. (2000). Controlling the environment to prevent suicide: International perspectives. *Canadian Journal of Psychiatry, 45,* 639–644.

Leenaars, A., Cantor, C., Connolly, J., EchoHawk, M., Gailiene, D., He, Z., et al. (2002). Ethical & legal issues in suicidology: International perspectives. *Archives of Suicide Research, 6,* 185–197.

Leenaars, A., Collins, P., & Sinclair, D. (2008, May 28). *Report to the London Police Service and London community on the deaths of David Lucio and Kelly Johnson.* Retrieved November, 22, 2008, from http://www.police.london.ca

Leenaars, A., DeLeo, D., Diekstra, R., Goldney, R., Kelleher, M., Lester, D., et al. (1997). Consultations for research in suicidology. *Archives of Suicide Research, 3,* 139–151.

Leenaars, A., de Wilde, E., Wenckstern, S., & Kral, M. (2001). Suicide notes in adolescents: A life-span comparison. *Canadian Journal of Behavioural Science, 33,* 47–57.

Leenaars, A., Fekete, S., Wenckstern, S., & Osvath, P. (1998). Suicide notes from Hungary and the United States. *Psychiatrica Hungarica, 13,* 147–159. [In Hungarian]

Leenaars, A., Girdhar, S., Dogra, T., Wenckstern, S., & Leenaars, L. (in press). Suicide notes from India and the United States: A thematic comparison. *Death Studies.*

Leenaars, A., Haines, J., Wenckstern, S., Williams, C., & Lester, D. (2003). Suicide notes from Australia and the United States. *Perceptual and Motor Skills, 92*, 1281–1282.

Leenaars, A., & Lester, D. (1994a). Suicide and homicide rates in Canada and the United States. *Suicide & Life-Threatening Behavior, 24,* 184–191.

Leenaars, A., & Lester, D. (1994b). Assessment and prediction of suicide risk in adolescents. In J. Zimmerman & G. Annis (Eds.), *Treatment approaches with suicidal adolescents* (pp. 47–70). New York: Wiley.

Leenaars, A., & Lester, D. (Eds.). (1996a). *Suicide & the unconscious.* Northvale, NJ: Aronson.

Leenaars, A., & Lester, D. (1996b). Gender and the impact of gun control on suicide and homicide. *Archives of Suicide Research, 2,* 223–234.

Leenaars, A., & Lester, D. (1997a). The impact of gun control on suicide and homicide across the life span. *Canadian Journal of Behavioural Science, 29,* 1–6.

Leenaars, A., & Lester, D. (1997b). The effects of gun control on the accidental death rate from firearms in Canada. *Journal of Safety Research, 28,* 119–122.

Leenaars, A., & Lester, D. (2001). The impact of gun control (Bill C-51) on homicide. *Journal of Criminal Justice, 29,* 287–294.

Leenaars, A., Lester, D., Baquedano, G., Cantor, C., Connolly, J., Ovuga, E., et al. (2009). Controlling the availability of the means of suicide—Restriction of access to drugs and medications. In D. Wasserman & C. Wasserman (Eds.), *The Oxford textbook of suicidology and suicide prevention: A global perspective* (pp. 574–576). Oxford, UK: Oxford University Press.

Leenaars, A., Lester, D., Lopatin, A., Schustov, D., & Wenckstern, S. (2002). Suicide notes from Russia and the United States. *Social and General Psychiatry, 12–3*, 22–28. [In Russian]

Leenaars, A., Lester, D., Wenckstern, S., & Heim, N. (1994). Suicide notes from Germany and the United States. *Suizidprophylaxe, 3*, 99–101. [In German]

Leenaars, A., Maltsberger, J., & Neimeyer, R. (Eds.). (1994). *Treatment of suicidal people.* London: Taylor & Francis.

Leenaars, A., Maris, R., & Takahashi, Y. (Eds.). (1997). *Suicide: Individual, cultural, international perspectives.* New York:Guilford.

Leenaars, A., Moksony, F., Lester, D., & Wenckstern, S. (2003). The impact of gun control (Bill C-51) on suicide in Canada. *Death Studies, 27,* 103–124.

Leenaars, A., Park, B., Collins, P., Wenckstern, S., & Leenaars, L. (in press). Martyrs' last letters: Are they the same as suicide notes? *Journal of Forensic Science.*

Leenaars, A., & Wenckstern, S. (1991). Suicide in the school-age child and adolescent. In A. Leenaars (Ed.), *Life span perspectives of suicide* (pp. 95–107). New York: Plenum.

Leenaars, A., & Wenckstern, S. (Eds.). (2004). Altruistic suicide: From sainthood to terrorism. *Archives of Suicide Research, 8,* 1–136.

Leong, F., & Leach, M. (Eds.). (2008). *Suicide among racial and ethnic minority groups.* New York: Routledge.

Lester, D. (1974). Demographic versus clinical prediction of suicidal behaviors. In A. Beck, H. Resnick, & D. Lettieri (Eds.), *The prediction of suicide* (pp. 71–84). Bowie, MD: Charles Press.

Lester, D. (1987). Murders and suicide: Are they polar opposites? *Behavioral Science & The Law, 5,* 49–60.

Lester, D. (Ed.). (1988a). *Why women kill themselves.* Springfield, IL: C. C. Thomas.

Lester, D. (1988b). Gun control, gun ownership and suicide prevention. *Suicide & Life-Threatening Behavior, 18,* 176–180.

Lester, D. (1988c). Restricting the availability of guns as a strategy for suicide prevention. *Biology & Society, 5,* 127–129.

Lester, D. (1992a). *Why people kill themselves* (3rd ed.). Springfield, IL: C. C. Thomas.

Lester, D. (1992b). Suicide in police officers: A survey of nations. *Police Studies, 15,* 145–147.

Lester, D. (1994). A comparison of fifteen theories of suicide. *Suicide and Life-Threatening Behavior, 24,* 80–88.

Lester, D. (1995). Preventing suicide in women and men. *Crisis, 16,* 79–84.

Lester, D. (2000). *Why people kill themselves: A 2000 summary of research on suicide.* Springfield, IL: Charles C. Thomas.

Lester, D., & Leenaars, A. (1993). Suicide rates in Canada before and after tightening firearm control laws. *Psychological Reports, 72,* 787–790.

Lester, D., & Leenaars, A. (1994). Gun control and rates of firearm violence in Canada and the United States. *Canadian Journal of Criminology, 36,* 463–464.

Lester, D., Perdue, W., & Brookhart, D. (1974). Murderers who have attempted suicide. *Psychological Reports, 35,* 238.

Lewinsohn, P., Garrison, C., Langhinrichsen, J., & Marsteller, F. (1989). *The assessment of suicidal behavior in adolescents: A review of scales suitable for epidemiological clinical research.* Rockville, MD: National Institute of Mental Health.

Lindsay, M., & Lester, D. (2004). *Suicide by cop.* Amityville, NY: Baywood.

Lindsay, M., & Lester, D. (2008). Criteria for suicide by cop incidents. *Psychological Reports, 102,* 603–605.

Litman, R. (1984). Psychological autopsies in court. *Suicide & Life Threatening Behavior, 14,* 188–195.

Litman, R. (1988). Psychological autopsies, mental illness and suicide intent. In J. Nolan (Ed.), *The suicide case* (pp. 69–82). Chicago: American Bar Association.

Litman, R. (1994). Responsibility and liability for suicide. In E. Shneidman, N. Farberow, & R. Litman (Eds.), *The psychology of suicide* (pp. 187–199). Northvale, NJ: Aronson.

Loo, R. (1984). Occupational stress in the law enforcement profession. *Canada's Mental Health, 1984, 32,* 10–13.

Loo, R. (1986). Suicide among police in a federal force. *Suicide & Life-Threatening Behavior, 16,* 379–385.

Loo, R. (1995, September). *Police suicide: Issues, prevention, and postvention.* Poster session presented at Work, Stress, and Health conference. Washington, DC.

Loo, R. (2001). Effective postvention for police suicide. *The Australian Journal of Disaster & Trauma Studies,* 2001–02, Retrieved October 2001, from http://www.massey.ac.nz/~trauma1

Loo, R. (2003). A meta-analysis of police suicide rates: Findings and issues. *Suicide & Life-Threatening Behavior, 33,* 313–325.

Los Angeles Board of Police Commissioners. (1997). Domestic violence in Los Angeles Police Department: How well does the Los Angeles Police Department police its own? *Report of the Domestic Violence Task Force. Office of Inspector General.* Los Angeles: Author.

Luborsky, L., McLellan, A., Woody, G., O'Brien, C., & Auerbach, A. (1985). Therapist success and its determinants. *Archives of General Psychiatry, 42*, 602–611.

Ludwig, J., & Cook, P. (2000). Homicide and suicide rates associated with implementation of the Brady Handgun Violence Protection Act. *Journal of the American Medical Association, 284,* 585–591.

Lund, L., & Smorodinsky, S., (2001). Violent death among intimate partners: A comparison of homicide and homicide followed by suicide in California. *Suicide & Life-Threatening Behavior, 31,* 451–459.

Lunde, D. (1975). *Murder and madness*. Stanford, CA: Stanford Alumni Association.

Lynn, T. (2002). Police suicide. *Law Enforcement Executive Forum, 2*(4), 173–185.

Maia, D., Marmar, C., Metzler, T., Naberge, A., Berger, W., Mendlowicz, M., et al. (2007). Post-traumatic stress symptoms in an elite unit of Brazilian police officers: Prevalence and impact on psychosocial functioning and on physical and mental health. *Journal of Affective Disorders, 97,* 241–245.

Malmquist, C. (1996). *Homicide: A psychiatric perspective*. Washington, DC: American Psychiatric Press, Inc.

Maltsberger, J. (1986). *Suicide risk: The formulation of clinical judgment*. New York: New York University Press.

Maltsberger, J. (2001). Grandiose fury. *Crisis, 22,* 144–145.

Maltsberger, J. (2002). Letters across the Pacific. *Crisis, 23*, 86–88.

Maris, R. (1981). *Pathways to suicide*. Baltimore: John Hopkins University Press.

Maris, R., Berman, A., & Silverman, M. (2000). *Textbook of suicidology*. New York: Guilford.

Maris, R., Berman, A., Maltsberger, J., & Yufit, R. (Eds.). (1992). *Assessment and prediction of suicide*. New York: Guilford.

Markush, R., & Bertolucci, A. (1984). Firearms and suicide in the United States. *American Journal of Public Health, 74,* 123–127.

Martin, G. (1998). Media influence to suicide: The search for solutions. *Archives of Suicide Research, 4*, 51–66.

Marzuk, P. (1989, April). *AIDS-related suicides.* Paper presented at the American Association of Suicidology conference, San Diego, CA.

Marzuk, P. (1994). Suicide and terminal illness. In A. Leenaars, J. Maltsberger, & R. Neimeyer (Eds.), *Treatment of suicidal people* (pp. 127–138). Hampshire, UK: Taylor & Francis.

Marzuk, P., Leon, A., Tardiff, K., & Nock, M. (2004). Suicide among police [Letter to the editor]. *American Journal of Psychiatry, 161,* 768.

Marzuk, P., Nock, M., Leon, A., Portera, L., & Tardiff, K. (2002). Suicide among New York police officers, 1977–1996. *American Journal of Psychiatry, 159,* 2069–2071.

Marzuk, P., Tardiff, K., & Hirsch, C. (1992). The epidemiology of murder suicide. *Journal of American Medical Association, 267,* 3179–3183.

Maxwell, S., Stolensky, D., Goodman, N., Sommers, P., & Boyd, J. (1984). Suicide by firearms. *New England Journal of Medicine, 310,* 46–49.

Medoff, M., & Magaddino, J. (1983). Suicides and firearm control laws. *Evaluation Review, 7,* 357–372.

Meichenbaum, D. (2005). 35 years of working with suicidal patients: Lessons learned. *Canadian Psychology, 46,* 64–72.

Menninger, K. (1938). *Man against himself.* New York: Harcourt, Brace & Co.

Mill, J. S. (1984). *Systems of Logic.* London: George Routledge. (Original published in 1892.)

Miller, L. (1998). *Shocks to the system: Psychotherapy of traumatic disability syndromes.* New York: Norton.

Miller, L. (2005). Police officer suicide: Causes, prevention and practical intervention strategies. *International Journal of Emergency Mental Health, 7,* 101–114.

Miller, L. (2006a). Suicide by cop: Causes, reactions and practical interventions. *International Journal of Emergency Mental Health, 8,* 165–174.

Miller, L. (2006b). *Practical police psychology: Stress management and crisis intervention for law enforcement.* Springfield, IL: Charles C. Thomas.

Miller, M., & Hemenway, D. (1999). The relationship between firearms and suicide: A review of the literature. *Aggression and Violent Behavior, 4,* 59–75

Milroy, C. (1998). Homicide followed by suicide: Remorse or revenge? *Journal of Clinical Forensic Medicine, 5,* 61–64.

Mohandie, K., & Hatcher, C. (1999). Suicide and violence risk in law enforcement: Practical guidelines for risk assessment, prevention, and intervention. *Behavioral Sciences and the Law, 17,* 357–376.

Mohandie, K., & Meloy, J. (2000). Clinical and forensic indicators of suicide by cop. *Journal of Forensic Sciences, 45,* 384–389.

Mohandie, K., Meloy, J., & Collins, P. (2009). Suicide by cop among officer-involved shooting cases. *Journal of Forensic Sciences, 54,* 456–462.

Mohandie, K., Piersol, F., & Klyver, N. (1996). Law enforcement turmoil and transitions and the evolving role of the police psychologist. In J. T. Reese & R. Solomon (Eds.), *Organizational issues in law enforcement* (pp. 383–396). Washington, DC: Federal Bureau of Investigation.

Möller, H.-J. (2001). Pharmacological treatment of underlying psychiatric disorders in suicidal patients. In D. Wasserman (Ed.), *Suicide and unnecessary death* (pp. 173–178). London: Martin Dunitz.

Morselli, E. (1882). *Suicide: An essay in comparative normal statistics.* New York: Appleton.

Mowat, R. (1966). *Morbid jealousy and murder.* London: Tavistock.

Mundt, D. (1990). Gun control and rates of firearm violence in Canada and the United States. *Canadian Journal of Criminology, 32,* 137–154.

Murphy, G. (1992). *Suicide in alcoholism.* New York: Oxford University Press.

Murray, H. (1938). *Explorations in personality.* New York: Oxford University Press.

Murray, H. (1967). Death to the world: The passions of Herman Melville. In E. Shneidman (Ed.), *Essays in self-destruction* (pp. 3–29). New York: Science House.

Narloch, R. (1973). *Criminal homicide in California.* Los Angeles, CA: California Department of Justice.

National Police Suicide Foundation. (2009). National P.O.L.I.C.E. suicide foundation. Retrieved January 11, 2009, from www.psf.org

Nolan, J. (1988). Suicide, sane or insane and suicidal intent. In J. Nolan (Ed.), *The suicide case* (pp. 51–65). Chicago: American Bar Association.

Oakland police shooting: The mourning after. (2009, March 23). *Oakland Tribune,* p. 1.

O'Connor, R., & Leenaars, A. (2004). A thematic comparison of suicide notes drawn from Northern Ireland and the United States. *Current Psychology, 22,* 339–347.

O'Connor, R., Sheeby, N., & O'Connor, D. (1999). A thematic analysis of suicide notes. *Crisis, 20,* 106–114.

Ogilvie, D., Stone, P., & Shneidman, E. (1969, March). Some characteristics of genuine versus simulated suicide notes. *Bulletin of Suicidology,* 17–26.

Palermo, G., Smith, M., Jentzen, J., Henry, T., Konicek, P., Peterson, G., et al. (1997). Murder-suicide of the jealous paranoid type: A multicenter statistical pilot study. *The American Journal of Forensic Medicine & Pathology, 18,* 374–383.

Palmer, S., & Humphrey, J. (1980). Offender-victim relationships in criminal homicide followed by offender's suicide. *Suicide & Life-Threatening Behavior, 10,* 106–118.

Palmer, B., Pankrantz, V., & Bostwick, J. (2005). The lifetime risk of suicide in schizophrenia: A re-examination. *Archives of General Psychiatry, 62,* 247–253.

Pam, E. (2001). Police homicide-suicide in relation to domestic violence. In D. Sheehan & J. Warren (Eds.), *Suicide and law enforcement* (pp. 357–363). Washington, DC: FBI.

Parent, R. (1998a). Victim-precipitated homicide. *RCMP Gazette, 60*(4), 2–14.

Parent, R. (1998b). Suicide by cop. *The Police Chief, 65*(10), 111–114.

Parolee stood over stricken police officers and fired again. (2009, March 22). *Oakland Tribune,* p. 1.

Peak, K., Gaines, L., & Glensor, R. (2004). *Police supervision and management in the era of community policing* (2nd ed.). Upper Saddle River, NJ: Prentice-Hall.

Perdue, W., & Brookhart, D. (1974). Murderers who have attempted suicide. *Psychological Reports, 35,* 238.

Pfeffer, C. (1986). *The suicidal child.* New York: Guilford.

Philips, D. (1974). The influence of suggestion on suicide: Substantive and theoretical implications of the Werther effect. *American Sociological Review, 39,* 240–253.

Philips, D. (1986, April). *Effects of the media.* Paper presented at the conference of the American Association of Suicidology, Atlanta, GA.

Pionaar, J., Rothmann, S., & van de Vijver, F. (2007). Occupational stress, personality traits, coping strategies, and suicide ideation in South African police services. *Criminal Justice and Behavior, 34,* 246–258.

Platt, S. (2007). Unemployment and suicidal behavior. *Social Science and Medicine, 19,* 93–115.

Powers, W. (1999). Confidentiality and counseling. *Personnel files, Chicago Police Department, 1*(2), 1.

Pritchard, C. (1996). Suicide in the People's Republic of China categorized by age and gender: Evidence of the influence of culture on suicide. *Acta Psychiatrica Scandinavica, 93,* 362–367.

Rainey, D., & Runyan, C. (1992). Newspapers: A source for injury surveillance? *American Journal of Public Health, 82,* 745–746.

Richman, J. (1991). Suicide and the elderly. In A. Leenaars (Ed.), *Life span perspectives of suicide* (pp. 153–167). New York: Plenum.

Richman, J. (1993). *Preventing elderly suicide*. New York: Springer.

Robinson, E. (1953). Richard Cory. In L. Thompson (Ed.), *Tilbury town: Selected poems of Edwin Arlington Robinson*. New York: Macmillan.

Rogers, C. (1951). *Client-centered therapy*. Boston: Houghton Mifflin.

Rosenbaum, M. (1990). The role of depression in couples involved in murder-suicide and homicide. *American Journal of Psychiatry, 147,* 1036–1039.

Roth, S. (2004). Suicide among police officers [Letter to the editor]. *American Journal of Psychiatry, 161,* 766–767.

Rourke, R., & Fisk, J. (1981). Socio-emotional disturbances of learning disabled children: The role of central processing deficits. *Bulletin of the Orthopsychiatry Society, 31,* 77–78.

Rourke, R., Young, G., & Leenaars, A. (1989). A childhood learning disability that predisposes those afflicted to adolescent and adult depression and suicide risk. *Journal of Learning Disabilities, 22*, 169–175.

Royal Commission on Aboriginal Peoples. (1995). *Choosing life: Special report on suicide among aboriginal people*. Ottawa: Ministry of Supply & Service.

Rudofossi, D. (2007). *Working with traumatized police officer-patients.* Amityville, NY: Baywood.

Satcher, D. (1998). Bringing the public health approach to the problem of suicide. *Suicide and Life-Threatening Behavior, 28,* 325–327.

Sayin, A., Leenaars, A., Candansayar, S., Akar, T., Demirel, B., & Leenaars, L. (2010). Different cultures, same reasons: A thematic comparison of suicide notes from Turkey and the United States. *Journal of Cross-Cultural Psychology*, 41, 253–263.

Schmidtke, A., Fricke, S., & Lester, D. (2001). Suicidal behavior among German police officers. In D. Sheehan & J. Warren (Eds.), *Suicide & law enforcement* (pp. 431–435). Washington, DC: FBI.

Second Mayerthorpe officer sues RCMP. (2009, March 18). *The Globe and Mail,* p. A8.

Selkin, J. (1976). Rescue fantasies in homicide-suicide. *Suicide & Life-Threatening Behavior, 6,* 79–85.

Selkin, J. (2005). *Suicide and the law: Cases, theories and strategies for prevention.* Buffalo, NY: William S. Hein & Co., Inc.

Sellbom, M., Fischler, G., & Ben-Porth, Y. (2007). Identifying MMPI-2 predictors of police officer integrity and misconduct. *Criminal Justice and Behavior, 34,* 985–1004.

Seltzer, J., Crockton, R., & Bartholomew, A. (2001). Psychiatric autopsies: Its use in police studies. In D. Sheehan & J. Warren (Eds.), *Suicide and law enforcement* (pp. 275–284). Washington, DC: FBI.

Shakespeare, W. (1952). Othello. In W. Clarke & W. Wright (Eds.), *The plays and sonnets of William Shakespeare* (pp. 205–243). Chicago: William Benton.

Shaughnessy, J., Zechmeister, E., & Zechmeister, J. (2000). *Research methods in psychology*. New York: McGraw-Hill.

Sheehan, D., & Warren, J. (Eds.). (2001). *Suicide & law enforcement.* Washington, DC: FBI.

Shneidman, E. (1963). Orientations toward suicide. In R. White (Ed.), *The study of lives* (pp. 200–227). New York: Atherton.

Shneidman, E. (1967). Sleep and self-destruction: A phenomenological approach. In E. Shneidman (Ed.), *Essays in self-destruction* (pp. 510–539). New York: Science House.

Shneidman, E. (1971). Perturbation and lethality as precursors of suicide in a gifted group. *Suicide & Life-Threatening Behavior, 1*, 23–45.

Shneidman, E. (1972). Foreword. In A. Cain (Ed.), *Survivors of suicide* (pp. ix–xi). Springfield, IL: Charles C. Thomas.

Shneidman, E. (1973). Suicide. In *Encyclopedia Britannica* (Vol. 21, pp. 383–385). Chicago: Williams Benton.

Shneidman, E. (1975). Postvention: Care of the bereaved. In R. Pasnau (Ed.), *Consultation-liaison psychiatry* (pp. 245–256). New York: Grune & Stratton.

Shneidman, E. (1977). The psychological autopsy. In L. Gottshalk (Ed.), *Guide to investigation and reporting of drug abuse deaths*. Washington, DC: U.S. Government Printing Office, US DHEW.

Shneidman, E. (1980). *Voices of death*. New York: Harper & Row.

Shneidman, E. (1981a). Psychotherapy with suicidal patients. *Suicide and Life-Threatening Behavior, 11*, 341–348.

Shneidman, E. (1981b). Postvention: The care of the bereaved. In E. S. Shneidman. *Suicide: Thoughts and reflections, 1960–1980* (pp. 157–167). New York: Human Sciences Press.

Shneidman, E. (1982). On "Therefore I must kill myself." *Suicide & Life-Threatening Behavior, 12*, 52–55.

Shneidman, E. (1984). Aphorisms of suicide and some implications for psychotherapy. *American Journal of Psychotherapy, 38*, 319–328.

Shneidman, E. (1985). *Definition of suicide.* New York: Wiley.

Shneidman, E. (1991). The commonalities of suicide across the life span. In A. Leenaars (Ed.), *Life span perspectives of suicide* (pp. 39–52). New York: Plenum.

Shneidman, E. (1993). *Suicide as psychache. A clinical approach to self-destructive behavior*. Northvale, NJ: Jason Aronson, Inc.

Shneidman, E. (1994). Clues to suicide reconsidered. *Suicide & Life-Threatening Behavior, 24*, 395–397.

Shneidman, E. (1999). On "Therefore I must kill myself." In A. Leenaars (Ed.), *Lives and deaths: Selections from the works of Edwin S. Shneidman* (pp. 72–76). Philadelphia: Brunner-Mazel.

Shneidman, E. (2001). Anodyne therapy: Relieving the suicidal patient's psychache. In H. Rosenthal (Ed.), *Favorite counseling and therapy homework assignments* (pp. 180–183). Philadelphia: Taylor & Francis.

Shneidman, E., & Farberow, N. (Eds.). (1957). *Clues to suicide*. New York: Harper & Row.

Shneidman, E., & Mandelkorn, P. (1967). How to prevent suicide. *Public Affairs Pamphlet No. 406.* New York: Public Affairs Committee.

Silverman, M., & Felner, R. (1995). The place of suicide prevention in the spectrum of intervention: Definition of critical terms and constructs. *Suicide & Life-Threatening Behavior, 25,* 10–21.

Slaby, A. (1992). Creativity, depression and suicide. *Suicide & Life-Threatening Behavior, 22*, 157–166.

Slaby, A. (1994). Psychopharmacotherapy of suicide. In A. Leenaars, J. Maltsberger, & R. Neimeyer (Eds.), *Treatment of suicidal people* (pp. 141–151). London: Taylor & Francis.

Slosar, J. (2001). The importance of perfectionism in law enforcement suicide. In D. Sheehan & J. Warren (Eds.), *Suicide and law enforcement* (pp. 539–547). Washington, DC: FBI.

Smith, K., Conroy, M., & Ehler, P. (1984). Lethality of suicide attempt rating scale. *Suicide & Life-Threatening Behavior, 14*, 215–242.

Smith, M., Glass, G., & Miller, T. (1980). *The benefits of psychotherapy*. Baltimore: Johns Hopkins University Press.

Sommers, P. (1984). The effects of gun control on suicide rates. *Atlantic Economic Journal, 12,* 67–69.

Stack, S. (1997). Homicide followed by suicide: An analysis of Chicago data. *Criminology, 35,* 435–453.

Stack, S. (1998). Research on controlling suicide: Methodological issues. *Archives of Suicide Research, 4,* 95–99.

Stahl, S. (2000). *Essential psychopharmacology*. Cambridge: Cambridge University Press.

Stengel, E. (1964). *Suicide and attempted suicide*. Baltimore: Penguin.

Stenger, E., & Stenger, E. (2000). Physical illness and suicidal behaviour. In K. Hawton & C. van Heeringen (Eds.), *Suicide and attempted suicide* (pp. 405–420). Chichester, UK: Wiley & Sons.

Stevenson, R., & Cox, G. (Eds.). (2008). *Perspectives on violence and violent death.* Amityville, NY: Baywood.

Stoff, D., & Mann, J. (Eds.). (1997). *The neurobiology of suicide: From the bench to the clinic.* New York: The New York Academy of Sciences.

Strupp, H., & Howard, K. (1992). A brief history of psychotherapy research. In D. Freedheim (Ed.), *History of psychotherapy* (pp. 309–334). Washington, DC: American Psychological Association.

Styron, W. (1990). *Darkness visible*. New York: Random House.

Sullivan, H. (1962). Schizophrenia as a human process. In H. Perry, N. Gorvell, & M. Gibbens (Eds.). *The collected works of Harry Stack Sullivan* (Vol. II). New York: W. W. Norton.

Sullivan, H. (1964). The fusion of psychiatry and social sciences. In H. Perry, N. Gorvell, & M. Gibbens (Eds.), *The collected works of Harry Stack Sullivan*. New York: W. W. Norton.

Task Force on Empirically Supported Therapy Relationships. (2001). *Empirically supported therapy relationships: Conclusions and recommendations of Division 29 task force.* http://www.academic.uofs.edu/faculty/NORCROSS/empir.htm

Thase, M., & Jindal, R. (2004). Combining psychotherapy and psychopharmacology for treatment of mental disorders. In M. Lambert (Ed.), *Bergin and Garfield's handbook of psychotherapy and behavior change* (5th ed., pp. 743–766). New York: John Wiley & Sons.

Thibault, E., Lynch, L., & McBride, R. (2004). *Proactive police management* (6th ed.). Upper Saddle River, NJ: Prentice-Hall.

Tomlinson-Keasey, C., Warren, L., & Elliot, J. (1986). Suicide among gifted women. *Journal of Abnormal Psychology, 95,* 123–130.

Toolan, J. (1981). Depression and suicide in children: An overview. *American Journal of Psychotherapy, 35,* 311–322.

Toynbee, A. (1968). Man's concern with death. In E. Shneidman (Ed.), *Death: Current perspectives.* Palo Alto, CA: Mayfield.

Turvey, B. (1995). Police officers: Control, hopelessness, & suicide. *Knowledge Solution—Campus.* Retrieved April, 1995, from http://www.corpus.delicit.com/suicide.html

Unnithan, N., Corzine, J., Huff-Corzine, L., & Whitt, H. (1994). *The currents of lethal violence.* Albany, NY: State University of New York Press.

U.S. Department of Health and Human Services. (2001). *National strategy for suicide prevention: Goals and objectives for action.* Rockville, MD: Author.

van der Wal, J. (1989,1990). The aftermath of suicide: A review of the empirical evidence. *Omega, 20,* 149–171.

van Praag, H. (1997). Some biological and psychological aspects of suicidal behavior: An attempt to bridge the gap. In A. Botsis, C. Soldatos, & C. Stefanis (Eds.), *Suicide: Biopsychosocial approaches* (pp. 73–92). Amsterdam: Elsevier.

Verkes, R., & Cowen, P. (2000). Pharmacotherapy of suicidal ideation and behaviour. In K. Hawton & K. van Heeringen (Eds.), *The international handbook of suicide and attempted suicide* (pp. 487–502). Chishester, UK: John Wiley & Sons.

Violanti, J. (1992). *Police retirement: The impact of change.* Springfield, IL: Charles C. Thomas.

Violanti, J. (1995, February). The mystery within: Understanding police suicide. *FBI Law Enforcement Bulletin,* 19–23.

Violanti, J. (2001). Police suicide: Current perspectives and future considerations. In D. Sheehan & J. Warren (Eds.), *Suicide and law enforcement* (pp. 437–446). Washington, DC: FBI.

Violanti, J. (2004a). Suicide among police officers. Letter to the editor. *American Journal of Psychiatry, 161,* 766.

Violanti, J. (2004b). Predictors of police suicide ideation. *Suicide & Life-Threatening Behavior, 34,* 277–283.

Violanti, J. (2007). Homicide-suicide in police families: Aggression full circle. *International Journal of Emergency Mental Health, 9,* 97–104.

Violanti, J., Vena, J., Marshall, J., & Petralia, S. (1996). A comparative evaluation of police suicide rate validity. *Suicide & Life-Threatening Behavior, 26,* 79–85.

Wampold, B. (1997). Methodological problems in identifying efficacious psychotherapies. *Psychotherapy Research, 7,* 21–43.

Wasserman, D. (2001, November). *The prevention of repeated suicide attempts.* Paper presented at the "No Suicide" International Congress, Geneva.

Watzlawick, P. (1976). *How real is real?* New York: Random House.

Watzlawick, P., Beavin, J., & Jackson, D. (1967). *Pragmatics of human communication.* New York: W. W. Norton.

West, D. (1966). *Murder followed by suicide: An inquiry carried out for the Institute of Criminology.* Cambridge, MA: Harvard University Press.

Wolff, H. (1931). Suicide notes. *American Mercury, 24,* 264–272.

Wolfgang, M. (1958). An analysis of homicide-suicide. *Journal of Clinical and Experimental Psychopathology, 19,* 208–218.

Wolfgang, M. (1959). Suicide by means of victim-precipitated homicide. *Journal of Clinical and Experimental Psychopathology, 20,* 335–349.

World Health Organization. (2002). *World report on violence and health*. Geneva: Author.

World Health Organization. (2006). *Preventing disease through healthy environments*. Geneva: Author.

Yalom, I., & Leiberman, M. (1971). A study of encounter group casualties. *Archives of General Psychiatry, 25,* 16–30.

Zelig, M. (1996). Workplace violence: The law enforcement setting. In J. T. Reese & R. Solomon (Eds.), *Organizational issues in law enforcement* (pp. 309–316). Washington, DC: Federal Bureau of Investigation.

Zilboorg, G. (1936). Suicide among civilized and primitive races. *American Journal of Psychiatry, 92,* 1347–1369.

Zilboorg, G. (1937). Considerations on suicide, with particular reference to that of the young. *American Journal of Orthopsychiatry, 7,* 15–31.

Index

SELECT TITLES FROM THE

Death, Value and Meaning Series

***Series Editor, Dale A. Lund** (former Series Editor: John D. Morgan)*

STEP INTO OUR LIVES AT THE FUNERAL HOME

Jo Michaelson

LOSS, GRIEF, AND TRAUMA IN THE WORKPLACE

Neil Thompson

A COP DOC'S GUIDE TO PUBLIC SAFETY COMPLEX TRAUMA SYNDROME
Using Five Police Personality Styles

Daniel Rudofossi

FREEDOM TO CHOOSE
How to Make End-of-Life Decisions on Your Own Terms

George Burnell

PERSPECTIVES ON VIOLENCE AND VIOLENT DEATH

Edited by Robert G. Stevenson and Gerry R. Cox

WORKING WITH TRAUMATIZED POLICE OFFICER-PATIENTS
A Clinician's Guide to Complex PTSD Syndromes in Public Safety Professionals

Daniel Rudofossi

SELECT TITLES FROM THE

Death, Value and Meaning Series

***Series Editor, Dale A. Lund** (former Series Editor: John D. Morgan)*

DEATH AND BEREAVEMENT AROUND THE WORLD
Volume 1: Major Religious Traditions

Edited by John D. Morgan and Pittu Laungani

DEATH AND BEREAVEMENT AROUND THE WORLD
Volume 2: Death and Bereavement in the Americas

Edited by John D. Morgan and Pittu Laungani

DEATH AND BEREAVEMENT AROUND THE WORLD
Volume 3: Death and Bereavement in Europe

Edited by John D. Morgan and Pittu Laungani

DEATH AND BEREAVEMENT AROUND THE WORLD
Volume 4: Death and Bereavement in Asia, Australia and New Zealand

Edited by John D. Morgan and Pittu Laungani

DEATH AND BEREAVEMENT AROUND THE WORLD
Volume 5: Reflective Essays

Edited by John D. Morgan, Pittu Laungani, and Stephen Palmer
